Deadly

How I safely switched to natural blood thinners

Ed Barker

Deadly Drug

I dedicate this book to Yvonne, my dear wife of 30 years,
who, together with Jesus Christ my Lord,
saved my life in June 2013

Disclaimer

The information in this book is not intended to replace a one-to-one relationship with a qualified health care specialist. The facts given here should not be interpreted as medical advice and are presented only for the sharing of information.

Nothing here should be taken as medical advice for dealing with any given problem, or to diagnose, treat, prevent or cure any disease. Consult your health-care professional for guidance on specific health issues.

The information in this book is a collection of facts that can be found in the public domain, and is presented for informational and educational use only. No claims can be made as to any benefits that might result from the use of information in this book.

Although I have made every effort to ensure this information is accurate and of a high standard, no warranties of any kind are made with regard to the completeness or accuracy of the content. The author disclaims any personal loss or liability caused or alleged to be caused, directly or indirectly, through the use of the information contained in this book.

All trademarks are property of their respective owners.

Contents

Introduction   11

1 How a blood clot almost killed me   19

2 Life in warfarin prison   25

3 Injecting dried pig mucous   33

4 A daily dose of rat poison   41

5 List of foods that can cause blood clots   57

6 Ten safe and effective natural blood thinners   73

7 Does your doctor know about this anti-clotting
   medical device?   95

8 A powerful (free) way to thin your blood naturally   99

9 What to do if you have factor V Leiden   107

10 Frequently asked questions   117

11 Side effects of five other blood-thinning drugs   125

About the author   133

Introduction

The doctor of the future will give no medicine,
but will educate his patients in the care of
the human frame, in diet, and in the cause
and prevention of disease.
(Thomas Edison)

In the UK, thousands of people each year develop a deep-vein blood clot. And many of those sufferers later die when it detaches from the vein wall and gets pumped to a lung artery, where it lodges and becomes a 'pulmonary embolism', blocking the flow of blood to the lungs. Deep vein thrombosis, which can lead to this life-threatening situation, is a serious health problem.

A 100,000-mile journey

The average adult body holds about 5 litres (9 pints) of blood, in constant movement through a flexible tube system of arteries, arterioles, capillaries, venules and veins. Our heart, which beats around 100,000 times a day, pumps oxygen-rich blood to the cells in our body. This blood eventually goes back to the heart via the veins, which then pumps it to our lungs so we can breathe out the toxic carbon dioxide in our blood. Next, fresh oxygenated blood from the lungs returns to the heart to start the whole process over again.

The tiniest blood vessels, capillaries, are usually about a third the thickness of a human hair. And a human adult has around 40 billion capillaries. To give an idea of how vast this number is, one billion is a thousand million. So, 40 billion is 40,000 million.

If all the blood vessels in an average adult were stripped out and laid in a straight line, the line would measure almost 161,000 kilometres (100,000 miles). A ball of string this long would wind around the earth's equator four times!

Astonishingly, our blood somehow manages to flow continuously through this 100,000-mile network of tubes. But it needs to move smoothly – a blockage anywhere in the vast network that forms this tube system, in the form of a blood clot, can result in severe disability, or even death.

Does your doctor always know what's best for you?

What does your doctor do if you develop a blood clot? He or she will prescribe you anti-clotting drugs to stop an existing clot from getting bigger and prevent new ones from forming. And these drugs do in fact work, but long-term use of drugs such as warfarin can also cause serious harm to your body. And not only that . . .

Because of the side effects of these drugs, your doctor may then prescribe further drugs to counteract the effects of the initial drugs prescribed. And these extra drugs also have side effects, which then need other drugs to counteract the new side effects. And so the medical merry-go-round whirls on – making boatloads of money for Big Pharma but leaving patients feeling depressed and trapped, unable to escape the daily routine of popping pills for fear of developing a new blood clot.

But how many warfarin takers know the more sinister side of this drug? More on this later.

So, we have doctors prescribing drugs such as warfarin that do some good in the short term, but also cause serious harm to the body if used for a long time, and are high-risk factors that may cause dangerous irreversible conditions – including *death*.

Medical doctors study only drugs-based medicine, doctors who are, in effect, the hands of Big Pharma, writing out one drugs prescription after another, week after week, year after year. And most doctors seem to have little interest in – and know little to nothing about – non-drugs-based alternatives that *cure* conditions rather than just *treat* them.

Safe anti-clotting alternatives

For lower-risk patients there are indeed safe and effective

long-term alternatives to potentially deadly anti-clotting drugs. These alternatives consist of (1) natural, plant-based substances without nasty side effects, (2) a little-known medical device, and (3) a powerful, ancient, free healing source. Keep reading and you'll get detailed information on the most effective clot-busting and blood-thinning natural remedies available. Remedies that help to heal and strengthen veins and arteries, and give your heart a new lease of life – and without any of the risky, crippling side effects of Big Pharma's drugs.

Who am I?

By this point you may be wondering about the author of this book. Who am I and what are my credentials to be writing about switching from warfarin to safer non-drug choices?

Simply this. I've had first-hand experience of this book's subject, and have done in-depth research on non-drug anti-clotting alternatives, information disclosed to you in later chapters of the book.

In June 2013 I had the shock of my life when I nearly collapsed on the side of the road, and a short time later found myself in an ambulance being rushed to the intensive care unit of our local hospital. What followed over the next six months led to my writing this book. Read on and you'll find out why, after researching the dangers of warfarin, I took myself off this deadly drug.

I'm a university graduate with a BA in psychology and English literature and a postgraduate teaching certificate. I used to be a school teacher: I taught GCSE English and English as a Second Language at a school in the UK. Then, in the late 1990s, I became a freelance copy editor, editing books for mainly academic UK and US publishers, which I've done on and off to the present, including some writing.

Why I jumped off the medical-pharmaceutical hamster wheel

When the doctor prescribed long-term warfarin for my deep vein thrombosis (DVT), this worried me greatly. I knew drugs have side effects, but at first knew nothing about the serious damage long-term warfarin use does to the body. The doctor mentioned no side effects and said nothing about my coming off this drug as soon as possible. (More on this later.)

Because I was unhappy about being a long-term warfarin slave, I began to research warfarin's harmful effects on the body. Shocked at what I uncovered, I began to search for safe natural alternatives. This book is the result of my experience with warfarin and my discovery of safe and effective non-drug alternatives.

When I was thinking of coming off warfarin, I felt vulnerable and nervous and had various questions:

• Is it safe to come off warfarin suddenly?

• What if another clot forms soon afterwards?

Are there safe, scientifically proven drug-free ways to keep my blood thin, so no more clots form and I avoid any further DVTs and pulmonary embolisms (PEs)?

• What about taking aspirin as a blood thinner – is it safe?

Perhaps you have the same questions. If so, this book may help you make some important choices about your own health. I've written it so you can get all the info you need in one handy place without having to spend days hunting around the Web for answers to your questions. Plus, at the end of each chapter I've included a 'References' section, so you can quickly check the facts for yourself, if you want to.

I've also tried to give the facts simply and briefly, so you don't have to plough through long blocks of text or struggle to understand complicated medical terms.

I'm writing this in December 2021, eight-and-a-half years since I nearly died from a DVT and PE, and I feel well and strong. I intend to continue using only natural proven alternatives to medical drugs to stay clot free and healthy. My daily, and then weekly, visits to the hospital to have often painful blood samples taken for analysis, and then the correct dose of warfarin prescribed, are now a distant memory. No more warfarin for me, ever.

It should take you just a few hours to read and digest the facts I've gathered here for you, where I lay out the steps I took to break free from warfarin. However, please note: patients in certain high-risk categories are advised to stay on warfarin for life (see the end of chapter 4). If you're in the lower-risk category and desperately want to escape

• constant blood monitoring
• being careful not to cut yourself
• worrying about how much dark-leaf veg you can eat

and switch instead to safe, natural clot-preventing alternatives, you'll know exactly what to do. Of course, I recommend you consult your doctor first – even though I did not – if you decide to launch out and take the natural, side-effect-free route. Taking yourself off warfarin is a big step and you need to make sure you have all the facts before making such a life-changing decision.

Once you've digested the information in this book, something else to bear in mind is that our human bodies vary from one another. We have different genetic make-ups and body types. A one-size-fits-all approach is not what this book is about. Here I've simply told you my story and the road I took, after doing some research, to freedom from warfarin and the Rockefeller–Carnegie medical system, set up in the early 1900s, that controls much of the way global health care works today.

If you decide to take the escape route I took, may you too experience the health and peace of mind I have today, eight-and-a-half years after saying goodbye to drugs-based medicine. Wishing you all the best for your own unique journey as you find your way safely through the medical-pharmaceutical minefield.

1

How a blood clot almost killed me

Also, when I walk through the
valley of the death-shadow,
I will fear no evil,
For You are with me.
(Holy Bible, Psalm 23:4)

Early danger signs

Around April 2013 I noticed the calf of my right leg starting to swell and become painful. Eventually it grew to around two-thirds wider than my left calf. Also, I noticed that when I walked briskly or climbed stairs I was getting more out of breath than normal. I wondered why this was, but did not think too much about it. I didn't go to a doctor, but let the situation continue for about three months.

Near collapse by the road

On 24 June 2013 my wife, Yvonne, went to visit a friend, Pam, who lived about half a mile from our house. I'd offered to drive around in the evening and pick Yvonne up from Pam's apartment.

Shortly before 10 pm I opened our garden gate and walked about 90 metres (100 yards) to our car, which was parked in the street. As I walked to the car, I was feeling very out of breath and slightly dizzy. Eventually, I reached the car and nearly fainted – I had to lean against the door to support myself.

I stood there for a while in the hope that the dizzy feeling would go away. It did after a few minutes and I got into the car to go and pick Yvonne up.

A short while later we returned. I parked the car and walked back to our house, but felt very unwell. I felt as if I might collapse at any moment.

When we were indoors, I told Yvonne I felt very unwell and asked her to call for an ambulance. Which she did. I felt myself fading away, and knew I could die at any moment. But I prayed to God that He would keep me in this life to look after Yvonne. After I'd prayed, I felt a bit better and came back to full alertness.

Rushed to Accident & Emergency

The ambulance people arrived within 15 minutes and did a health check on me with some kind of machine. I was surprised though that their check took as long as it did, because I still felt very ill and believe I could have died before they got me to hospital.

After talking to me and finishing all their tests, about half an hour after the ambulance had arrived, the crew decided to take me to the Accident & Emergency (A&E) section of our local hospital, just a few minutes' drive away. Yvonne was very worried and sat with me in the back of the ambulance.

When we got to the A&E a doctor spoke to me and asked what had happened and how I was feeling. The upshot was that he diagnosed me as having had a *heart attack*, and around *6 o'clock the following morning* the hospital staff transferred me to the hospital's Acute Cardiac Unit. (*Note*: I'd experienced no pain in my heart area!) Yvonne was exhausted, as she'd sat with me throughout the night, and went home by taxi so she could get some rest.

Hospital experience – ups and downs

For the next four days I experienced what it was like to be a hospital patient. The last time I'd stayed in hospital was 53 years before, when I was 2 years old – to have my tonsils removed. The nurses were kind and efficient, and I have only good things to say about them. Likewise, with the doctors and other medical staff who attended to our needs within the ward. But the hospital food left a lot to be desired. It was very unhealthy – a lot of sugary, high-carbohydrate stodge.

Side note: during my stay in hospital, one of the other patients had a hospital nutritionist come to see him. I overheard part of the conversation. The nutritionist advised the skinny patient to eat lots of *sausage rolls*, as they are 'healthy food'. I couldn't believe my ears. What kind of advice was this, from a supposed health professional, for someone recovering from a serious illness? Sausage rolls have little to no nutritional value at all.

Apart from the unhealthy food, it was fairly difficult to sleep in the hospital bed at night, owing to how noisy the ward was and the bright lights. But Yvonne kindly brought me some ear plugs and a face mask so I could cover my eyes and block out the annoying light.

I was there for four days.

Apart from the awful food, the stay wasn't too bad. I had some interesting conversations with other patients, who were bed-bound in the same ward as I, and used the time to have a good rest. Strangely, though, at no time during those four days did they scan my swollen leg. As mentioned earlier, the doctor first diagnosed me as having had a heart attack. But what about the leg?

Medications

After being in the heart ward for three days I was moved to the pulmonary (lung) ward – the doctors had rediagnosed me as having had a blood clot, a deep vein thrombosis (DVT), in my swollen leg. The clot had detached from the vein's wall, broken into smaller clots, known as 'emboli', which my blood had then swiftly shot to my lungs.

As mentioned above, this condition is known as a pulmonary embolism (PE).

These clots in the lungs had caused my breathlessness and, I discovered later, could have killed me. A study reported in the medical journal *Experimental & Clinical Cardiology* says that acute PE, if untreated, leads to death in 30 per cent – around a third – of cases.

Getting back to the hospital stay. While I was there, the doctor prescribed two drugs for my condition – heparin, a liquid, and warfarin tablets. Heparin prevents new clots from forming and also prevents existing clots from getting larger. Warfarin, on the other hand, keeps the blood from clotting too quickly – it slows down the clotting process, known as the 'clotting cascade'.

The heparin had to be injected into my stomach every evening, which was a nasty experience. Also, had I known then what was in heparin, I would have been a lot more cautious about self-injecting it into my stomach after leaving the hospital (more on this later).

Warfarin came in the form of small blue, pink and brown tablets, a combination of which I had to take once a day. Again, had I known then what I was putting into my body every time I swallowed these tablets, I would have stopped taking them far sooner than I did.

In the next chapter I'll briefly describe what life was like for the two months I injected myself in the stomach with heparin, and the six months I was on warfarin.

Perhaps you've had the same rocky ride and may, once you've read this book, written after many hours of research, weigh up the pros and cons and decide to take the exit I took.

References

http://www.nhs.uk/conditions/Anticoagulants-warfarin-/Pages/Introduction.aspx (accessed 6 June 2017)

http://www.gosh.nhs.uk/medical-information-0/medicines-information/warfarin (accessed 6 June 2017)

http://www.ouh.nhs.uk/patient-guide/leaflets/files/100429warfarinchildren.pdf (accessed 6 June 2017)

http://www.med.unc.edu/htcenter/patient-care/clotting-disorders/blood-clot-education-1/how-are-blood-clots-treated (accessed 6 June 2017)

https://www.ncbi.nlm.nih.gov/pmc/articles/PMC3718593 (accessed 10 December 2021)

https://medlineplus.gov/druginfo/meds/a682826.html (accessed 10 December 2021)

2
Life in warfarin prison

*The greatest prison in the
universe is an ignorant mind.
(Matshona Dhliwayo)*

When you go to your doctor with a health issue, he or she usually gives you a drug prescription. The online *Oxford Dictionary* defines a 'drug' as 'A medicine or other sub-stance which has a physiological effect when ingested or otherwise introduced into the body.'

In my case, because I'd had a DVT in my calf, which had broken up into smaller clots and shot to my lungs, my doctor prescribed heparin injections and warfarin tablets. The heparin injections were a short-term solution – to prevent any new blood clots from forming, or existing ones from growing larger – and had to be stopped when my blood was clotting at the correct rate. By taking the right combination of warfarin tablets I could keep this clotting rate consistent.

The problem is, once you start travelling the pre-scription-drug route you're dependent on these drugs to keep your medical condition manageable – drugs do not *cure* a condition, but only keep it stable and manageable. It's not in Big Pharma's interests to cure you, but to keep you coming back for more. They want a constant flow of repeat customers, which is what these drugs supply. The sicker you are and the more drugs you become dependent on, the more money Big Pharma makes. Shocking, but true. Few realize how the current medical system works – it's far more about profit than about health.

Daily jabbing the needle into my stomach

After being discharged from the pulmonary unit at our local hospital, I picked up my prescription for heparin injections and warfarin tablets. Then followed around two months of painful daily injections of the heparin solution into my stomach. I had to do these injections myself, and it was a horrible experience. Plus, I had to inject myself at the same time each day, which was difficult if I was out and about.

What I didn't know then, but found out only four years later when doing research for the first edition of this book is what heparin is made of. Perhaps you'll be as disgusted as I was when you read what I discovered (see chapter 3). Had I known then what I now know about the source of heparin, I would have stopped injecting myself with it soon after coming out of the hospital.

'I can't find the vein!'

As with any drug, you have to take warfarin in the correct amounts. Swallow too much, and it thins your blood to dangerous levels. Take too little, and your blood clots too fast – which heightens your risk of further blood clots clogging a vein and turning into a pulmonary embolism.

To make sure I took the correct dose of warfarin, I had to trek to our local hospital at first daily and then later once a week to have blood sucked out of a vein into a syringe. The hospital visit was a pain, in more ways than one.

First, Yvonne (who kindly usually came with me) and I had to find a free parking space in a road as near to the hospital as possible. Hospital parking is expensive and we tried to avoid having to pay these costs. Also, we didn't know how long we'd have to wait before the person taking the blood sample called for me. The longer we waited, the more expensive the parking would be.

Once in the 'phlebotomy' (the blood-sampling) section, I had to take a ticket and join the queue. After a while the phlebotomist would call my name and I'd go into her cubicle (it was usually a woman). She'd then ask me to extend my arm while she tried to find a vein before sticking the needle in to suck out some blood. Most of the time when I made these visits to have a blood sample taken, the person drawing the blood gave me a not-too-painful experience. It depended on who was doing the procedure. But sometimes the phlebotomist couldn't find a vein, and struggled to get a vial of blood.

One woman, an American, invariably gave me a painful experience when I had the misfortune to be called by her. Every time I visited the hospital to have blood drawn, I prayed someone else would do the task. Perhaps she'd had too little training? Or she just didn't like me? Who knows? Whatever the reason, I didn't look forward to my weekly hospital visit.

Having said that, I was grateful to be living in the UK, where there was at least a medical system in place that dealt with various health crises in a reasonably efficient way. (However, at the time of my writing this, 2022 is almost upon us, and I now do my best to stay away from doctors, hospitals or anything to do with the medical establishment.)

Usually the next day after my hospital visit I received a notification in the post from the hospital stating what dosage of warfarin I should take to keep my blood-clotting rate within safe levels.

'Don't forget to take your warfarin'

So, not only did I have to remember to inject myself daily with the heparin solution, but I also had to take the right dose of warfarin, and at the same time of day. Plus, always having to remember to take the warfarin tablets with me when I went out could be a nuisance. And then, having to take them at the same time of day, in the evening, was another restriction. Moreover, there were the dietary no-nos.

'Don't eat too much spinach!'

While taking warfarin I felt I was constantly walking a dietary tightrope, doing a daily balancing act regarding what warfarin-affecting foods I could eat and in what quantities. No cranberry juice or too much green leafy veg, for example, because these could interfere with warfarin's anti-clotting action.

On the subject of cranberry juice and warfarin the May/June 2006 issue of the *American Journal of Therapeutics* reported:

> We encountered a patient taking stable doses of warfarin who developed major bleeding and high INR [international normalized ratio, a measure of how fast the blood clots] soon after starting daily cranberry juice.
>
> No other identifiable reasons for the high INR were apparent.
>
> The patient resumed his usual dose of warfarin after stopping the juice. This case suggests a definite relationship between cranberry juice and warfarin.

So, if you're on warfarin and enjoy a glass of cranberry juice, the drink is definitely off limits.

Likewise, while on warfarin, you'll have to be careful about how much broccoli, spinach and kale you eat, as all of these have high levels of vitamin K, the vitamin responsible for helping your blood to clot. Warfarin reduces the effectiveness of vitamin K in the body, so your blood stays thinner than it would otherwise. If you eat too many helpings of green leafy veg, your vitamin K level shoots up. But moderate helpings of leafy vegetables are all right.

A 2008 article on clotcare.com states, 'It is a common misconception that people on warfarin should avoid vitamin K . . . Rather than avoiding vitamin K, you should maintain a consistent intake of vitamin K by maintaining a consistent diet.' In other words, from week to week, you should eat the same types of foods. (See chapter 9 for lists of foods high in vitamin K.) Keep your diet consistent, and the amount of vitamin K in your body stays relatively stable, which helps you take the right amount of warfarin to keep your blood from clotting too fast. *But how easy is it to eat consistently?*

'Don't cut yourself while shaving!'

Another huge warfarin lifestyle restriction is that you have to be careful not to cut yourself when you shave (if you're a male). Or do you like to chop your own vegetables in the kitchen? Then watch out – a slip of that sharp chopping knife could be fatal! And don't blow your nose too hard, because you could have a nosebleed. Once you're on warfarin your blood stays thin and won't clot easily – your nose could bleed and bleed and bleed . . .

Side note: if you cut yourself while shaving or cut a finger, there's a quick and easy way to stop the bleeding. Simply slightly dampen a black tea bag (green tea will also work) and push it firmly on to the cut. Maxillofacial (to do with the jaws and face) surgeon Dr Bonine says tea contains tannic acid, which helps to form blood clots.

Although your veins and arteries are a blessing when sealed, puncture a vein or artery wall and you face a serious problem if you're on warfarin: getting your blood to clot, so the break in your blood vessel gets sealed and you don't bleed to death. Prevention is easier than cure, so you have to be careful to avoiding puncturing your body in any way.

No more contact sport or cycling

Do you enjoy contact sport, such as rugby or riding your bike? Then you have to set these activities aside while you're on warfarin. Those who take part in certain sports are vulnerable to injury, which can lead to serious, unstoppable blood flow.

Imagine cycling and being involved in a collision with a car. Or if a dog runs out in front of you and you swerve to avoid it and smash into a wall. Once you start bleeding, it's tough to stop the flow. And if you're unconscious, those attending you may not know you're on blood-thinning warfarin – they won't know how to deal effectively with your situation. *What a stressful way to live!*

Is there a way out?

Because of all these restrictions – 'Don't . . .', 'Don't . . .', 'Don't . . .' – for me it sometimes felt like being in 'drug prison'. First heparin, and then warfarin had taken control of large parts of my life and I wanted to be free of their ugly grip. Six months on warfarin felt far too long, and I wanted out. However, before we investigate the warfarin alternatives, in the next chapter we look at what heparin contains and its possible dangerous side effects.

References

http://journals.lww.com/americantherapeutics/Abstract/2006/05000/Warfarin_Cranberry_Juice_Interaction_Resulting_in.17.aspx (accessed 9 June 2017)

http://www.clotcare.com/vitaminkandwarfarin.aspx (accessed 9 June 2017)

https://www.drbonine.com/stop-bleeding.html (accessed 14 December 2021)

3
Injecting dried pig mucous

There is nothing more
daring than ignorance.
(Menander)

What is heparin?

Heparin, also known as dalteparin, marketed under the name Fragmin® by the pharmaceutical company Pfizer, Inc., is an injectable liquid to stop existing blood clots from getting bigger, and to prevent new ones forming in the veins. But where does heparin come from?

Perhaps you'll be as astonished as I was to find out that this widely used anti-clotting agent comes from the mucous of *pig intestines*, which is dried and then turned into powder. Yes, you read that correctly: heparin comes from pig intestines.

And these intestines are processed to a large extent on farms in China. The 10 October 2016 issue of the *Chemical & Engineering News* magazine has an article with the title 'Making heparin safe'. The article says:

China's huge pig population is the reason why the country is a superpower when it comes to making heparin, an anticoagulant used around the globe during heart surgery and dialysis as well as for the treatment of deep vein thrombosis. The country accounts for half of the world's heparin production.

Pig intestine mucosa is currently the only approved raw material for producing the heparin sold in most of the world, including the U.S. And given that each mucosa yields only a few grams of heparin, China's huge pig population is essential to the world's supply of the drug.

When you inject yourself with this anti-clotting drug, you may well be squirting into your body dried mucous that comes from a pig farm in China. But what else does heparin contain, and what does this have to do with human health?

Should these chemicals be in your body?

The medicines.org.uk website, apart from the heparin itself, lists six other substances that act as the vehicle or medium for the drug. This is what your typical heparin solution consists of, and what you put into your body each time you inject yourself with this liquid:

• Benzyl alcohol
• Methyl hydroxybenzoate (E218)

- Sodium citrate dihydrate
- Sodium chloride
- Water for injections

Let's take a look at the first five in the list.

Benzyl alcohol, says the toxnet.nlm.nih.gov website, is

> used in a wide variety of products including
> photographic developer for color movie films;
> dyeing nylon filament, textiles, and sheet plastics;
> solvent for dyestuffs, cellulose esters, casein,
> waxes; heat-sealing polyethylene films; inter-
> mediate for benzyl esters and ethers; bacterio-
> static; cosmetics, ointments, emulsions; ball point
> pen inks; stencil inks.

This same web article says benzyl alcohol is a known skin irritant and can cause an allergic reaction in some people.

Methyl hydroxybenzoate (E218), says the *British Journal of Pharmacology*, is used as a preservative in drugs and food. It increases shelf life, so products stay usable for a greater length of time.

Propyl hydroxybenzoate (E216), says the ukfoodguide.net website, is a preservative found in many cosmetics. It is also used to preserve drugs and food. The website says children should avoid this substance.

According to the European Commission website, methyl hydroxybenzoate and propyl hydroxybenzoate may each 'cause allergic reactions (possibly delayed), and exceptionally, bronchospasm'.

Taking sodium citrate into your body, says the livestrong.com website, can lead to

> uncontrolled muscle spasms and contractions . . .
> It could result in muscle tears or bone fractures . . .
>
> Because of this possibility, if you are taking sodium citrate, contact your physician if you notice sudden muscle pain or uncontrolled contractions of the hand or foot muscles.

Sodium chloride is another name for table salt. This, with the other ingredients that make up a drug, is commonly added to water to form a solution ready for injection into a vein.

More heparin side effects

The drugs.com website lists the following among the possible side effects a heparin injection may cause:

• bleeding from the gums when brushing teeth
• coughing up blood
• dizziness
• severe or continuing headaches

• sudden nosebleeds

• vomiting up blood or a substance that looks like coffee grounds

And even after a patient stops using heparin, the following side effects may occur:

• severe sudden headaches

• sudden loss of coordination

• sudden slurred speech

• sudden vision changes

Under a subheading about the most important fact to know about dalteparin, a type of heparin, the drugs.com website says:

> Dalteparin can cause a very serious blood clot around your spinal cord if you undergo a spinal tap or receive spinal anesthesia (epidural), especially if you have a genetic spinal defect, a history of spinal surgery or repeated spinal taps, or if you are using other drugs that can affect blood clotting, including blood thinners or NSAIDs [non-steroidal anti-inflammatory drugs] (ibuprofen, Advil, Aleve, and others).
> This type of blood clot can lead to long-term or permanent paralysis.

Get emergency medical help if you have symptoms of a spinal cord blood clot such as back pain, numbness or muscle weakness in your lower body, or loss of bladder or bowel control.

In the next chapter we move on to look at some of the disturbing facts on warfarin, the other anti-clotting drug many doctors still prescribe. We also investigate why, after examining the facts, you might decide to come off this drug as fast as possible.

References

http://cen.acs.org/articles/94/i40/Making-heparin-safe.html (accessed 9 June 2017)

https://www.medicines.org.uk/emc/medicine/8308 (accessed 9 June 2017)

https://toxnet.nlm.nih.gov/cgi-bin/sis/search/a?dbs+hsdb:@term+@DOCNO+46 (accessed 9 June 2017)

https://www.ncbi.nlm.nih.gov/pmc/articles/PMC1572324 (accessed 9 June 2017)

http://www.ukfoodguide.net/e216.htm (accessed 9 June 2017)

https://ec.europa.eu/health/sites/health/files/files/eudralex /vol-2/c/guidelines_excipients_july_2013_rev_1.pdf (accessed 9 June 2017)

http://www.livestrong.com/article/315235-sodium-citrates-side-effects (accessed 9 June 2017)

4
A daily dose of rat poison

What is food to one, is
to others bitter poison.
(Lucretius, De Rerum Natura*)*

Warfarin – an interesting history

In North America and Canada in the 1920s cattle started to bleed very easily, even from minor cuts. What caused this bleeding? It was the food these cattle were eating – silage made from sweet clover.

Sweet clover contains coumarin, a substance that stops blood from clotting at its normal rate. But it was not until 1940 that the scientists Karl Link and Harold Campbell found out the identity of the anti-blood-clotting compound in sweet clover: 4-hydroxy coumarin. Then, in 1948, Link made the first batch of warfarin, a name derived from WARF (Wisconsin Alumni Research Foundation) and 'arin' from coumarin.

Warfarin got the green light in 1952 to be used as rat poison, and in 1954 for use as a human anticoagulant.

Keeps humans alive but kills rats?!

Why is warfarin so effective as a rat poison? Well, rats are cautious about what they eat. Any whiff of poison and they scamper off in disgust. Also, they eat only small amounts at a time, so they need to keep eating before the poison builds up inside them and causes them to bleed internally, which kills them. The ideal rat poison has to be odourless and then be combined with the kind of food rats love: cereal. The rat tucks into its favourite food, now mixed with warfarin, and blissfully munches away, until it eventually keels over.

But how can something that kills rats be helpful to humans? This is the question I asked myself when I discovered that warfarin is a rat poison, and began seeking natural anti-clotting alternatives.

What's in each warfarin tablet?

About five months after getting on the warfarin treadmill I started to research the contents of this drug. Inspecting the information insert that came with the warfarin, I noticed that one of warfarin's ingredients is 'aluminum lake'. This set my alarm bells ringing, as 'aluminum' is the US word for 'aluminium', and I knew aluminium has a deadly effect on the human brain. Think dementia . . .

A 2012 article in naturalnews.com states that aluminum lake is a food colouring that contains 'dangerous amounts of aluminum and harmful synthetic petrochemicals. These "petrochemicals" are carcinogens containing petroleum, antifreeze and ammonia, which cause a long list of adverse reactions.' Petroleum, antifreeze and ammonia?

The article goes on to say that 'Aluminum poisoning can lead to short and long term central nervous system (CNS) damage, such as memory impairments, autism, epilepsy, mental retardation, and dementia.'

Furthermore, the newswise.com website reports on a study by the Intermountain Healthcare Clinical Pharmacist Anticoagulation Service in Salt Lake City, USA. The study, over a period of seven years and completed in 2016, looked at 10,537 patients without any history of dementia. These patients were all on warfarin, and the study director, Dr T. Jared Bunch, says, 'Our study results are the first to show that there are significant cognitive risk factors for patients treated with Warfarin over a long period of time.' He also says, '[O]nly those that absolutely need blood thinners should be placed on them long-term.'

So what else do the blue, pink, brown and white warfarin tablets contain? Holding your breath?

The medicines.org.uk website, in a May 2017 update, lists the following ingredients of a 0.5, 1, 3 or 5 milligram warfarin tablet:

• warfarin sodium

• anhydrous lactose

• pregelatinized maize starch

- quinoline yellow (E104; 1 mg only)
- erythrosine (E127; 5 mg only)
- allura red (E129; 1 mg and 5 mg)
- indigotine (E132; 1 mg and 3 mg)

As we did for the injectable heparin solution, let's look at each of the above ingredients in turn.

Warfarin sodium is the active ingredient of each tablet, the substance that prevents the blood from clotting (and causes rats to bleed to death).

Anhydrous lactose is made up of two sugars: glucose and galactose. It is 'anhydrous' because all the water has been removed. Because it's a sugar it makes an ideal coating for pills – it helps improve a pill's taste. However, the livestrong.com website says, 'If you are lactose intolerant and consume lactose, you may develop gas, diarrhea, bloating or abdominal pain.' So those with a lactose intolerance may experience discomfort after taking warfarin tablets.

Pregelatinized maize starch is a starch that has been dried and then cooked. In an article on modified corn (maize) starch the healthwyze.org website says:

> These modified starches are difficult for a body to digest, and of course, there have been no publicly-released studies about the long-term effects of eating these mystery substances from the chemical industry.

Modified corn starch often contains about 10% maltodextrin, which is a common keyword used by industry to hide the presence of mono-sodium glutamate.

Dr Joseph Mercola, on his mercola.com website, des-cribes monosodium glutamate (MSG) as a 'silent killer that's worse for your health than alcohol, nicotine and many drugs'. Citing the highly respected neurosurgeon Dr Russell Blaylock, Mercola says MSG 'overexcites your cells to the point of damage or death, causing brain damage to varying degrees – and potentially even triggering or worsening learning disabilities, Alzheimer's disease, Parkinson's disease, Lou Gehrig's disease and more'.

Now, for the next ingredient: magnesium stearate. Magnesium stearate, a salt that results when magnesium ions bond with stearic acid, is a powder added to tablets to stop them sticking to each other. It's also used as a bulking agent, to make the tablet fuller than it would otherwise be. In a web article entitled 'Stop Using Magnesium Stearate .. . Go Organic!' Mike Masci, President of Ingredient Evo-lution, lists some of the reasons why it's safer to steer clear of magnesium stearate.

He says it comes mainly from genetically modified plant sources such as cottonseed oil, rapeseed oil and palm oil. Genetically modified plants have been shown to be harmful for human consumption. Plus, a 2007 study showed that tablets containing magnesium stearate are not absorbed as easily in the stomach juices as tablets that have no magnesium stearate in them.

Masci goes on to cite a 2009 Japanese study that showed magnesium stearate in tablets can cause formaldehyde to form in the body. Interestingly, the study says lactose in tablet form, another component of warfarin tablets, also generates formaldehyde. Why is this a problem?

Because formaldehyde, used in embalming fluid, according to a TIME magazine web article, is 'an extremely nasty substance that can cause irritation in the eyes and breathing problems in human beings at elevated levels'. The article says Canada declared formaldehyde a toxic substance in 1999, and the International Agency for Research on Cancer says it's a cancer-forming agent. While the amounts of toxic, cancer-forming formaldehyde warfarin tablets might generate in the short term are tiny, how much would a long-term warfarin user absorb into his or her body?

The final items on the list of warfarin tablet ingredients are the colourings quinoline yellow (E104; 1 mg tablet only), allura red (E129; 1 mg and 5 mg tablets), erythrosine (E127; 5 mg tablet only) and indigotine (E132; 1 mg and 3 mg tablets).

Quinoline yellow, a food colouring added to scotch eggs, smoked haddock and ice cream, says the ukfoodguide.net website, heightens hyperactivity in children. This was a finding of Southampton University in the UK. This colouring is banned in many countries, including the USA, Australia, Japan and Norway, but not in the UK.

Allura red also causes hyperactivity in children say the researchers from Southampton University and can cause cancer in mice. This dye is added to sweets and drinks to give them an orangey red colour. Among the countries that have banned its use are Switzerland, France, Germany, Austria, Sweden, Denmark and Norway. The ndhealth-facts.org website adds that allura red is added to some cosmetics.

Erythrosine is a pink or red dye made from coal tar. It's added to cocktail, glacé or tinned cherries, and to tinned fruit, biscuits, salmon spread, paté and custard mix, among others. When food is processed above 200 degrees centigrade, erythrosine releases iodide, which could affect the thyroid gland, leading to hyperthyroidism – over-activity of the thyroid gland. A 1990 study showed that hyperthyroidism causes cancer in rats. This food additive is banned in the USA and Norway, but not in the UK.

As for indigotine, the ukfoodguide.net website des-cribes it as a 'blue synthetic coal tar dye, normally produced by a synthesis of indoxyl by fusion of sodium phenylglycinate in a mixture of caustic soda and soda-mide'. Indigotine is added to tablets and capsules. Used in some ice creams, sweets and biscuits, it can cause a skin rash, itching, high blood pressure and breathing problems, and is banned in Norway. Children, especially, should not consume this dye.

Now, what other kinds of deadly effects can the chemical concoction in warfarin tablets have on the human body?

Ten possible warfarin side effects

Below I list just ten warfarin side effects, gleaned from a number of reputable medical websites. These are just the tip of the iceberg, as there are *many more* warfarin side effects than those listed below!

1 Excessive bleeding, which is difficult to stop

On his website heartmdinstitute.com, American cardiologist (heart specialist) Dr Stephen Sinatra says of warfarin that it 'has the dubious distinction of topping the list of medication-related emergency hospitalization for seniors. In my cardiology practice, I was always wary of blood thinning medications and used them with considerable caution, as of course would any doctor.' He says bleeding may occur if a patient swallows too much warfarin.

Male warfarin users have to be especially careful when shaving that they don't cut themselves. Bleeding gums as a result of vigorous teeth brushing is another common problem of warfarin patients. Or blowing your nose too hard can lead to a nosebleed.

2 Blurred vision

3 Slurred speech

4 Fits

5 Loss of consciousness

6 Purple toes

7 Gangrene and possible limb amputation

8 Yellowing skin and whites of the eyes (indicating possible liver problems)

9 Skin death (necrosis)

10 Hair loss (alopecia)

But *long-term* warfarin users should also be aware of other serious health problems warfarin can cause.

Three more warfarin side effects you may not know about

The three warfarin side effects I've listed below for you are rarely mentioned. Just these three alone would persuade me to stay well away from warfarin, unless my medical condition forced me to stay on this drug, as coming off it might be too risky.

1 Artery calcification

Long-term warfarin use causes hardening of the arteries, which in turn leads to heart disease. Our bodies need vitamin K1, an important factor in getting the blood to clot correctly. But we also need vitamin K2, which causes our bodies to use calcium correctly so it doesn't stick to our artery walls and over time calcify them.

So how does warfarin cause a problem?

The body needs vitamin K1 in order to produce vitamin K2. But warfarin blocks vitamin K1, so the body can't produce vitamin K2. The calcium in our blood has no way to be directed to where it is meant to go, and instead sticks to the inside of the arteries, eventually blocking them as more and more calcium lodges in these tiny tubes. The US National Library of Medicine National Institutes of Health website says 'Vitamin K plays a role in coagulation, and deficiency may promote coronary artery calcification'.

But the lack of vitamin K2 in the body, due to warfarin use, over time causes another serious problem – osteoporosis.

2 Osteoporosis (hardening of the bones, so they become brittle and break easily)

In the absence of vitamin K2, there is no way for the calcium to be steered into the bones and teeth; thus strengthening them. Eventually the bones become weak and break easily. This is especially the case with the backbones, forearms and hips.

American cardiologist Dr John Day says the Japanese, possibly because of their high intake of vitamin K2 (in, for example, the fermented soybean natto), have very low rates of bone fractures.

3 Liver damage

Although rare, warfarin can also damage the liver. The livertox.nih.gov website says that typically 'acute liver injury arises within 3 to 8 weeks of starting warfarin'. And overdosing on warfarin 'can result in excessive bleeding and hepatic [liver] failure'.

The hindawi.com website reports the case of a 64-year-old woman who died from the effects of warfarin on her liver. The autopsy showed that more than 90 per cent of her liver was 'replaced by tumor masses'.

As warfarin use can be deadly, are there safe alternatives?

In this chapter I've laid out some of the dangers associated with warfarin (including its use as a rat killer). The question is, do patients prescribed warfarin *have* to stay on it, or are there *safe, natural alternatives* to this drug? I tackle this subject in chapters 6 and eight.

Keep reading and you too may decide to replace warfarin with a safe alternative, assuming you don't fall into any of the high-risk categories heart expert Dr Stephen

Sinatra lists on his heartmdinstitute.com. Under the heading 'Who Should Stay on Coumadin [warfarin]?' Sinatra says patients in the following situations are 'often recommended' to stay on warfarin:

- Hearts with enlarged chambers or valves that don't work properly.
- Had a massive heart attack; the resulting scar tissue can weaken the left ventricle and allow blood to clot easier.
- Prosthetic or mechanical heart valves, or a pacemaker; blood is likelier to stick to the artificial surfaces.
- Had an embolic stroke (one of three kinds of strokes, where a piece or the whole clot of blood goes from the heart to the brain).
- Experienced atrial fibrillation, where the heart beats irregularly; blood can form pools and thicken.

He says diabetics and people prone to blood clots should stay on warfarin.

Weighing up heparin and warfarin use – pros and cons

As both heparin and warfarin can cause serious side effects, is it a good idea to use these drugs in the long term? Having done in-depth research on both drugs and the alternatives I describe in chapters 6 and 8, my view is this (again please note, I'm not giving medical advice, but just stating my personal opinion).

In an *emergency* DVT and PE situation it makes sense to follow the medical-drug route. But after the doctors have dealt with the emergency, what options are there for patients in the lower-risk group? Such patients might consider coming off these drugs as soon as possible, and replacing them with safe natural alternatives that have no known side effects on the human body.

If, like me, you don't like the thought of injecting dried pig mucous into your stomach or swallowing rat poison once a day long term to avoid further dangerous blood clots, then please keep reading.

Side note: if you like what you've read so far in this book and have found it to be helpful, please *leave a review that says how the book has helped you*. I'd greatly appreciate it. Thanks!

References

http://www.naturalnews.com/10-Artificial-Food-Coloring-Petroleum-Based-Industrial-Chemicals.html (accessed 9 June 2017)

http://www.newswise.com/articles/view/652707/?sc=dwhr &xy=10005670 (accessed 9 June 2017)

https://www.medicines.org.uk/emc/PIL.27631.latest.pdf
(accessed 9 June 2017)

http://www.livestrong.com/article/446556-what-is-anhydrous-lactose (accessed 9 June 2017)

http://healthwyze.org/reports/261-understanding-foods-labeled-modified-what-is-modified-food-starch-and-should-it-be-avoided (accessed 9 June 2017)

http://www.naturalnews.com/034813_childrens_medicines_aluminum_pills.html (accessed 12 June 2017)

http://www.newswise.com/articles/view/652707/?sc=dwhr&xy=10005670 (accessed 12 June 2017)

https://www.medicines.org.uk/emc/medicine/27651#EXCIPIENTS (accessed 12 June 2017)

https://www.medicines.org.uk/emc/PIL.27631.latest.pdf
(accessed 12 June 2017)

http://healthwyze.org/reports/261-understanding-foods-labeled-modified-what-is-modified-food-starch-and-should-it-be-avoided (accessed 12 June 2017)

http://articles.mercola.com/sites/articles/archive/2009/04/2
1/msg-is-this-silent-killer-lurking-in-your-kitchen-
cabinets.aspx (accessed 12 June 2017)

http://healthland.time.com/2011/06/11/why-the-federal-
government-finally-acted-on-chemical-safety (accessed
12 June 2017)

http://ukfoodguide.net/e104.htm (accessed 12 June 2017)

http://www.ukfoodguide.net/e127.htm (accessed
12 June 2017)

http://ukfoodguide.net/e129.htm (accessed 12 June 2017)

http://www.ndhealthfacts.org/wiki/Food_Colourings
(accessed 12 June 2017)

http://www.ukfoodguide.net/e132.htm (accessed
12 June 2017)

https://heartmdinstitute.com/heart-health/prescription-
blood-thinners-caution (accessed 24 May 2017)

https://www.ncbi.nlm.nih.gov/pubmed/27061505
(accessed 12 June 2017)

http://drjohnday.com/category/vitamin-k2 (accessed 26 May 2017)

https://livertox.nih.gov/Warfarin.htm (accessed 12 June 2017)

https://www.hindawi.com/journals/cricc/2016/7389087 (accessed 12 June 2017)

https://heartmdinstitute.com/heart-health/coumadin-warfarin (accessed 30 May 2017)

5
List of foods that can cause blood clots

It is easier to change a man's religion
than to change his diet.
(Margaret Mead)

O ne of the main ways to avoid developing a blood clot is to cut out certain types of food. Foods can either benefit or harm us, and below I give you a list of foods that may cause blood clots.

But first we must look at the area of 'inflammation'.

Inflammation causes blood clots

The word 'inflammation' comes from the Latin *inflammare,* which means 'into flame'. When part of your body becomes swollen or hot it is said to be inflamed.

Inflammation is your body's protective response to invading bacteria, viruses or toxic chemicals. When one of these enemies enters your body, your immune system activates cells that trap them and begin to heal damaged tissue. This can lead to pain, swelling of the affected area, redness or bruising.

There are two types of inflammation: *acute* and *chronic.* Acute inflammation lasts just a short time, and may be a response to, say, a splinter in your finger or a cut. Chronic inflammation, on the other hand, lasts much longer. This takes place when your immune system sends out cells that attack the body itself, such as in rheumatoid arthritis, where the joint tissues are constantly damaged.

Blood clots result when a chemical reaction takes place in your blood, changing your blood from a liquid to a solid. This happens when the fibrinogen in your blood is changed to fibrin, as happens when a scab forms over a cut in your finger. In his book *Over-the-Counter Natural Cures,* pharmacist Shane Ellison says:

> The molecule that controls this life-saving process is known as thromboxane. It not only heals but also saves us from bleeding to death. Like Glen Canyon Dam holds in the waters of Lake Powell, thromboxane is essential for keeping our blood where it belongs – within the 100,000 miles of veins, arteries, and capillaries. But if thromboxane elicits the formation of a clot within narrowed, inflamed arteries, the once-harmless clot becomes a death sentence. (P. 59)

Ellison goes on to say that inflammation is the root cause of blood clots. When our arteries become inflamed, this triggers the thromboxane which forms blood clots that clog the arteries – leading to a heart attack or stroke. He also says, 'being obese is a huge disservice to the health of your cardiovascular system. Obesity causes inflammation. And inflammation can switch on your blood-clotting cascade. Particularly, being overweight raises the levels of thromboxane' (p. 70).

So, if inflammation is the main cause of blood clots, it stands to reason that we should try to avoid as far as possible foods that cause inflammation in our bodies. But what are the main examples of such foods?

Eight foods that cause blood clots

Below I list eight foods you should steer clear of if you want to stay healthy and keep your inflammation levels optimal. Remember, inflammation can result in blood clots, so it's wise to avoid foods that contain substances that cause inflammation.

1 Sugar

Table sugar and high-fructose corn syrup are often added to foods in the West. Researchers found that sugar can cause inflammation to the cells that line the inside of blood vessels. Sugar can also cause obesity, diabetes and cancer. So, it's important to keep your sugar intake as low as possible.

The Cleveland Clinic says the average American eats around a whopping seventeen teaspoons of sugar a day. No more than six teaspoons or, better still, none, is a far healthier level.

2 Trans fats

Trans fats are vegetable oils that have hydrogen added to them. This makes the oils solid at room temperature and lengthens their shelf life.

According to the Mayo Clinic (online article 'Trans Fat Is Double Trouble for Your Heart Health'):

> Trans fat is considered the worst type of fat you can eat. Unlike other dietary fats, trans fat – also called trans-fatty acids – raises your 'bad' cholesterol and also lowers your 'good' cholesterol.
>
> A diet laden with trans fat increases your risk of heart disease, the leading killer of adults. The more trans fat you eat, the greater your risk of heart and blood vessel disease.
>
> Trans fat is so unhealthy that the Food and Drug Administration has recently prohibited food manufacturers from adding the major source [hydrogenated oils?] of artificial trans fat to foods and beverages.

Examples of foods that contain trans fats – which should be eaten as little as possible, or never – are as follows:

• cakes, biscuits and pies
• shortening

- microwave popcorn
- pizza
- fried foods, such as french fries, doughnuts and fried chicken
- non-dairy coffee creamer
- margarine

The Mayo Clinic article goes on to say, 'Trans fat, particularly the manufactured variety found in partially hydrogenated vegetable oil, appears to have no known health benefit. Experts recommend keeping your intake of trans fat as low as possible.'

3 Red and processed meat

In his online article 'The Top 10 Inflammatory Foods to Avoid' Dr Thomas Ball lists red and processed meat. He says researchers at the University of California San Diego School of Medicine found a molecule in red meat that may cause a permanent inflammatory response in the meat eater's body. This 'low-grade, simmering inflammation' may lead to cancer and heart disease.

Dr Ball also says processed meat – meat that has been smoked, cured or preserved with chemicals – can cause cancers of the colon, rectum, oesophagus and lungs. Meat of this type includes, for example, hot dogs, ham, corned beef and sausages. While we don't have to avoid red meat completely, 'No amount of processed meat is safe.'

4 Mono-sodium glutamate (MSG)

This substance, made from fermented starch or sugar, is added to food to heighten the food's flavour. Often found in soups, processed meats, Asian food and soy sauce, it is also in many products on supermarket shelves.

The authors of a 2008 study recorded in the *Journal of Autoimmunology* reported that MSG injected into mice causes 'significant inflammation' and suggested MSG 'should have its safety profile re-examined and be potentially withdrawn from the food chain'.

When you check a food label to see what that food contains, be aware that the following are other names for MSG or foods that produce glutamic acid:

- natural flavouring
- seasoning
- spices
- barley malt
- malt extract
- maltodextrin
- textured protein
- textured vegetable protein
- protein isolate
- protease
- pectin (E440)
- carrageenan (E407)

- hydrolyzed vegetable protein
- autolyzed yeast
- autolyzed yeast protein
- glutamic acid
- calcium glutamate
- hydrolyzed yeast
- yeast extract
- soy extracts
- bouillon/broth/stock

5 Artificial sweeteners

If you look at the list of ingredients on the back of a can of diet drink, or on the wrapper of a bar of chewing gum, the chances are you'll see the artificial sweetener aspartame mentioned. Or it may be called by one of these names:

Acesulfame potassium (K)

Canderel®

NutraSweet®

NutraSweet New Pink

AminoSweet®

Neotame®

Equal®

Blue Zero Calorie Sweetener Packets™

Advantame®

Pal Sweet Diet®

But what is this sweetener and why is it so dangerous? Believe it or not, according to a upi.com 'Science News' article aspartame is made in a laboratory from the faeces (waste products) of genetically modified Ecoli bacteria. After you put it into your mouth, it breaks down into phenylalanine, methanol and aspartic acid. Methanol is a type of alcohol that, when stored at high temperatures, breaks down into formaldehyde, which is highly toxic in the human body. (Formaldehyde, also found in electronic vaping cigarettes, is one of the components of embalming fluid!)

It is believed aspartame was one of the contributors to the Gulf War syndrome that afflicted thousands of US troops during the Gulf War conflict. These troops drank large amounts of diet drinks that had sat in cans in the scorching Middle Eastern sun. The aspartame in these drinks would have broken down into methanol and formaldehyde long before the soldiers quenched their thirst with this deadly, toxic brew.

Among the over ninety-two symptoms aspartame causes are the following:

- bulging eyes
- tinnitus (a buzzing sound in the ears)
- epileptic seizures
- migraines

- confusion
- numbness of the limbs
- tremors
- severe depression
- heart palpitations
- abdominal pain
- itching
- asthma
- hair loss
- irreversible brain damage
- birth defects
- multiple sclerosis
- suicidal tendencies
- death

To stay clot-free it is essential you avoid this dangerous chemical that causes massive inflammation in the human body. Although banned in Romania since the early 1990s, aspartame is legal for public use in the USA and UK.

6 Wheat

Scientists have found that amylase-trypsin inhibitors (ATIs), a group of proteins in wheat, can trigger serious inflammation affecting the kidneys, lymph nodes spleen and brain. ATIs can also worsen rheumatoid arthritis, multiple sclerosis, asthma and lupus, among other conditions.

These proteins are also found in gluten, another component of wheat and other grains. Researchers have shown that gluten too can cause inflammation in the human body.

As wheat, and grains generally, can trigger severe inflammation, it is best to exclude them from your diet if possible.

7 Oils

Omega-6 oils are also implicated in causing inflammation – over-consumption of these can cause the body to produce pro-inflammatory chemicals. Examples of foods rich in omega-6 oils, which should be avoided if possible, are as follows:

• corn

• safflower

• sunflower

• soybean

• cottonseed

• peanut

• sesame

• rapeseed (similar to canola)

On the topic of rapeseed oil, used in many products in the UK, the Bio-Pesticides DataBase of the University of Hertfordshire says this oil is used as a pesticide to control 'a range of sucking and chewing insects', such as mites, spidermites and mealybugs. Rapeseed oil is an *insect pesticide* added to much of the food on supermarket shelves!

The blog Smart Holistics in their article 'The Dark Side of Rapeseed Oil' says, 'mention is rarely made of the very toxic substance rapeseed oil also contains [erucic acid]. Not only does it irritate mucous membranes, but damages the myelin sheath around nerves and interferes with the use of Vitamin E by the body.'

The blog goes on to say that although new strains of rapeseed with lower amounts of erucic acid have been developed (notably canola oil), these genetically modified strains are still dangerous to human health. They can weaken blood vessels and cause cardiovascular disease, as well as developing plaques in the brain, a contributor to Alzheimer's disease. Plus, these genetically modified rapeseed oils have been linked to cancer, diabetes and obesity.

The Smart Holistics blog also says the rapeseed oil on supermarket shelves is not cold-pressed, but has been subjected to heat and chemicals in a factory. This process creates harmful transfats, which have been linked to assorted health problems.

A 1992 study mentioned in the *Journal of Thrombosis and Haemostasis* found that men fed a diet high in sunflower oil and another diet high in low-erucic acid rapeseed oil had a greater amount of blood platelet clumping (which can lead to blood clots) than when these men were fed a diet high in milk fat.

It is safer to major on foods high in omega-3 oils, which promote good health and do not stoke up inflammation, such as the following:

- salmon
- mackerel
- sardines
- oysters
- trout
- herring
- halibut
- cod liver oil
- flaxseeds
- pumpkin seeds

8 Refined carbohydrates

Before the twentieth century people tended to eat fibre-rich foods such as unprocessed seeds, fruits and roots. However, when food started to be mass produced, much of its fibre was removed – think white bread, for example.

The benefits of fibre are that it makes us feel full, helps to keep our blood sugar in check and provides food for our gut bacteria.

Food that has the fibre stripped out, however, is high in carbs and spikes our blood sugar. It also causes inflammation in the gut and, as we have seen, inflammation is a major risk factor in developing blood clots.

Foods high in refined carbs include the following:

• jam (jelly)
• chutney
• honey
• sweets (candy)
• refined cereals
• bread
• biscuits (cookies)
• cakes
• pastries
• pasta
• white flour

Conclusion

In order to live a clot-free life we have to monitor what we eat. If a certain type of food is high on the list of inflammation-triggering foods, it is wise to abstain from that food. Replacing, say, slices of white bread and jam with a piece of grilled salmon and salad will help to lower the amount of inflammation exploding in our bodies.

But we don't need to starve ourselves or go on a monk's diet. All we should do is *replace the bad foods with good ones.* After all, no one pours mud into the fuel tank of their car. Why treat our bodies – which are far more important than a car – any differently?

References

Ellison, S., *Over-the-Counter Natural Cures*, Naperville: Sourcebooks Inc., 2009

https://www.ncbi.nlm.nih.gov/books/NBK279298 (accessed 15 November 2021)

https://www.arthritis.org/health-wellness/healthy-living/nutrition/foods-to-limit/8-food-ingredients-that-can-cause-inflammation (accessed 16 November 2021)

https://www.webmd.com/arthritis/about-inflammation (accessed 1 December 2021)

https://my.clevelandclinic.org/health/symptoms/21660-inflammation (accessed 16 November 2021)

https://pubmed.ncbi.nlm.nih.gov/18508964 (accessed 16 November 2021)

https://www.mayoclinic.org/diseases-conditions/high-blood-cholesterol/in-depth/trans-fat/art-20046114 (accessed 16 November 2021)

https://www.webmd.com/diet/high-glutamate-foods#1 (accessed 16 November 2021)

https://performancehealthcenter.com/2020/02/the-top-10-inflammatory-foods-to-avoid (accessed 15 November 2021)

https://pubmed.ncbi.nlm.nih.gov/18178378 (accessed 16 November 2021)

https://www.prevention.com/food-nutrition/a20472934/other-names-for-msg (accessed 16 November 2021)

https://foodsthathealyou.com/over-34-hidden-names-for-msg (accessed 16 November 2021)

https://www.upi.com/Science_News/2013/08/26/Aspartame-patent-reveals-E-coli-feces-used/8131377527919 (accessed 9 December 2021)

https://draxe.com/nutrition/aspartame (accessed 17 November 2021.

https://www.ourgom.com/aspartame (accessed 17 November 2021.

https://www.medicalnewstoday.com/articles/313514 (accessed 17 November 2021)

https://www.smartholistics.co.uk/news-blog/the-dark-side-of-rapeseed-oil (accessed 29 November 2021)

https://openheart.bmj.com/content/openhrt/6/1/e001011.full.pdf (accessed 29 November 2021)

https://www.thieme-connect.de/products/ejournals/abstract/10.1055/s-0038-1648446 (accessed 29 November 2021)

https://www.nia.nih.gov/health/what-happens-brain-alzheimers-disease (accessed 11 December 2021)

6
Ten safe and effective natural blood thinners

Nature heals. The doctor's task consists in strengthening the natural healing powers, to direct them, and especially not to interfere with them.
(Hippocrates, c. 460–375 BC)

Just to clarify, at the start of this chapter, what I mean by 'blood thinners'. These are substances that keep the blood from clotting too quickly. They do not make the blood thinner, as if you were diluting it. 'Blood thinners' has become a common term for 'anti-clotting-agents', also known as 'anticoagulants'.

The four blood thinners I've listed for you below are just a few of the natural remedies that fight irregular blood-clot formation.

1 Nattokinase, from a popular Japanese food

Nattokinase is an enzyme taken from natto, fermented soybeans. The Japanese have eaten natto for over 1,000 years, and today eat around 7.5 billion packets of natto per year. Some researchers believe this food is the reason why there is so little heart disease in Japan, even though the Japanese are among the world's heaviest smokers. Statistics have shown that the Japanese live longer than anyone else on the planet – the men on average to around 78, and the women to 85.

But how does nattokinase melt away blood clots? It dissolves the fibrin in the blood. Fibrin is a meshlike substance that forms when a blood vessel gets a hole in its wall. The fibrin turns into a clot which then plugs the hole and stops the blood from leaking out.

Japanese scientist Hiroyuki Sumi discovered nattokinase in 1980 while working at Chicago University Medical School. He was interested in the clot-dissolving abilities of 137 natural foods. Dropping some natto into an artificial blood clot created in the laboratory, he left the natto there at a temperature close to that of a normal body. Within 18 hours the Natto had completely dissolved the clot. Sumi had made a remarkable discovery, and named the clot-dissolving enzyme he had found 'nattokinase', meaning 'natto enzyme'.

To date, at least seventeen scientific studies have been carried out on nattokinase. Respected natural health practitioner Dr David Williams, in a web article titled 'Nattokinase: The Japanese Clot-Busting Miracle', says that when blood flow in a blood vessel is restricted, or a clot forms, conventional medicine's answer is ultra-expensive 'clot-busting' drugs like streptokinase, activase, and urokinase.

These drugs are administered within minutes after a heart attack or stroke because their fibrin-olytic activity (ability to dissolve clots and the fibrin deposits that cause clots) lasts for only 4 to 20 minutes.

A far more effective natural solution for removing fibrin deposits is found in the Japanese soybean-based food natto.

In the same article he says that Japanese researchers have found that 100 grams (3.5 ounces) of natto have the same clot-dissolving power as a urokinase injection. But where-as the effects of the urokinase last between 4 and 20 minutes, those of the natto last up to 8 hours.

Dr Williams adds, 'Nattokinase is one of the most significant tools for improving chronic circulation prob-lems I have uncovered in the last several years.' American heart specialist Dr Stephen Sinatra also sings the praises of nattokinase. He says:

One of my top recommendations to lower your blood pressure naturally is with a nutrient called nattokinase, which comes from the Japanese food natto.

I like the fact that it addresses an often overlooked problem that causes high blood pressure to develop: hyperviscosity.

In other words, it helps to counteract thick, sick, sticky, and inflamed blood – keeping your blood flowing as it should.

I still take nattokinase most days and credit this to be one of the reasons why I have not developed any further blood clots in the eight years since I had a DVT and PE.

2 Krill oil, gift of the ocean

Krill are shrimplike creatures found in the open ocean. They vary in size from 8 millimetres to 60 millimetres (about 1/4 inch to 2 inches) and are an important food source for whales, fishes and birds. These tiny marine animals live in huge swarms either near the surface of the ocean or at depths as great as 2,000 metres (around 6,600 feet). In the Antarctic ocean, swarms of krill can be as dense as 20 kilograms per cubic metre (around 35 pounds per cubic yard).

Many natural health professionals recommend the use of fish oils to benefit heart health, including keeping the blood healthy, so as to avoid blood clots. However, krill oil is far superior to fish oils.

Both krill oil and fish oil contain omega-3 fats, which help to prevent blood clots forming. But as much as 50 per cent of the fish oil supplements on the market are of little use. The main reason is that fish oil oxidizes easily – when it comes into contact with oxygen, it degrades and loses its health-promoting benefits.

When health expert Dr Moerck conducted tests on krill oil and fish oil, he found that fish oil went rancid after just 1 hour's exposure to oxygen. The krill oil, however, took 190 hours' exposure to oxygen to go rancid, making it hugely more beneficial than fish oil.

Well-known American health guru Dr Joseph Mercola recommends eating only wild Alaskan salmon, because most ocean fish, and especially the larger ones such as tuna, are now contaminated with mercury, which is highly toxic to the human body. However, with krill oil, he says, 'your risk of getting any mercury contamination is extremely low' because 'krill are so small they don't have the chance to accumulate toxins before being harvested'. Mercola himself takes krill oil every day.

The cleanmarinekrill.co.uk website also says krill oil is preferable to fish oil. The body absorbs krill oil 59 per cent easier than it does fish oil, which means just one small capsule a day of krill oil does the work of a much larger dose of fish oil.

A number of clinical trials have shown that the health benefits of krill equal those of fish oil regarding heart health, brain function and joint health, but at far smaller doses. Also krill oil contains the powerful anti-oxidant astaxanthin, lacking in fish oil.

Dr Mercola reports a study where subjects took 12 milligrams (0.0004 ounces) of astaxanthin per day for eight weeks. At the end of this time, the subjects had a 20 per cent decrease in a protein that indicates heart disease. He says this protein 'is essentially an indicator of systemic inflammation in your body, and lower levels tend to be associated with a reduced risk of not only heart disease but many other chronic health problems as well'.

Mercola cites other studies that prove the benefits of astaxanthin, which

- improves blood flow
- lowers blood pressure
- decreases the oxidation of cholesterol that aids the build-up of arterial plaque

So, krill oil is preferable to fish oil and makes a valuable addition to the list of effective natural blood thinners.

3 Garlic, a powerful natural health aid

The garlic plant is part of the onion, chive and leek family. Native to central Asia, it also grows wild in parts of Europe. People have eaten garlic as a health food and medicine since ancient times. The Chinese used it as one of their most popular health remedies as long ago as 2,700 BC. And the ancient Egyptians gave it to their slaves to keep them strong, healthy and thus able to work harder. Plus, before major battles Greek generals fed their armies garlic.

The *Journal of Nutrition,* in a 2001 article titled 'Historical Perspective on the Use of Garlic', says athletes in the ancient Olympic Games ate garlic as a 'performance enhancer' before competing in the games. Roman naturalist and army commander Pliny the Elder (AD 23–79), a friend of the emperor Vespasian, used garlic as a general remedy. In the Byzantine Empire in the ninth century AD people ate garlic to prevent blood vessels from ageing. German doctors treated soldiers with garlic during the First World War, and the Russian army used garlic as an antibiotic.

Garlic is also a powerful anti-clotting agent. An article published in the *Pharmacognosy Review Journal* in 2010 says garlic decreases the fattiness of the blood. Because of this,

> garlic reduces the risk of atherosclerosis, whereby it prevents depositing of lipids [fats] in blood vessels.
>
> People from countries that often use garlic in their cuisine are less susceptible to blood vessel diseases, especially atherosclerosis [hardening of the arteries].

The article says garlic has been shown to have a powerful 'antithrombotic action'.

According to a research paper published in the *African Journal of Biotechnology* in 2008:

> A great deal of research has been completed and published on the anticoagulant and anti-thrombotic activities of garlic (*Allium sativum*).
>
> The beneficial effects of garlic include lowering of plasma cholesterol, decrease of fibrinogen, coupled with increased fibrinolytic activity, and inhibition of platelet activity.
>
> Platelets are tiny cell-like structures in blood that clump together and are involved in forming a blood clot.

The paper goes on to say:

> The inhibitory effect of processed garlic on human platelet aggregation [clumping together] has been known since 1978 (Lawson et al., 1992).
>
> According to Mohammad and Woodward (1986), when an aqueous [water-based] extract of garlic was added to platelet rich plasma (PRP), platelet aggregation was inhibited.

These findings clearly showed that garlic has anticoagulant properties.

4 Pine bark extract keeps the blood from clotting

The bark of the European coastal pine, apart from its other health-promoting benefits, has been shown to have blood-thinning properties.

One of the supplements made from pine bark extract, Pycnogenol®, prevented smoking-induced clotting in 19 American smokers, according to a 1999 study reported on the greenmedinfo.com website. Quoting the *Thrombotic Research* journal that published the study, the website says, 'This study showed that a single, high dose, 200 mg Pycnogenol, remained effective for over 6 days against smoking-induced platelet aggregation [clumping].'

In another article on the same website, titled 'How Pine Bark Extract Could Save Air Travelers Lives', the writer describes a 2004 study. This study looked at the anti-clotting effects of Pycnogenol® on air travellers. The travellers took Pycnogenol® a few hours before their flight, 6 hours after flying, and the day after flying.

In the control group, which received no Pycnogenol®, there was one deep vein thrombosis as a result of flying, and four minor blood clots. But the subjects who took Pycnogenol® stayed clot free.

The writer of the greenmedinfo.com article quotes the study's conclusion: 'Pycnogenol treatment was effective in decreasing the number of thrombotic events (DVT and SVT) in moderate-to-high risk subjects, during long-haul flights.' A 2005 study showed that Pycnogenol® taken before a flight and then 6 hours after the start of the flight greatly reduced the risk of ankle swelling, which is linked to deep vein thrombosis.

5 Curcumin, the golden spice

Curcumin is the part of turmeric that gives the spice its yellow colour. And it is the curcumin that has anti-clotting properties – it slows down the blood platelets sticking together and thus prevents blood clots. It also lowers inflammation, which is a major cause of deep vein thrombosis (see chapter 5).

In the study 'Anticoagulant Activities of Curcumin and Its Derivative', published in 2012 in the journal *BMB Reports*, researchers found that curcumin prevents blood clots, and suggest that eating turmeric daily may help to keep a person free from developing blood clots.

Because curcumin keeps the blood platelets from clumping together, it helps the blood flow more easily through tiny blood vessels known as microcapillaries. This increased blood flow increases the amount of oxygen and nutrients that reach the tissues, which aids in keeping us healthy.

A 2019 study reported in the journal *Phytotherapy Research* showed that curcumin also improves the flexibility of arteries, which helps the blood flow better and improves heart health. According to Dr Randy Baker, a holistic medicine practitioner of forty years, turmeric is one of the most health-promoting herbs around.

6 Bromelain, gift of the pineapple

Known as the 'queen of fruits', pineapple is not only delicious, but also has medicinal properties. It contains a proteolytic enzyme called bromelain, which is found in the juice, but mainly in the stem and core of the pineapple. An enzyme is a substance a living organism produces that causes a biochemical reaction, and a proteolytic enzyme is an enzyme that breaks proteins and peptides (two or more linked amino acids that form a chain) down into simple amino acids.

Bromelain is a powerful blood-clot preventer. Unlike nattokinase, which dissolves blood clots, bromelain is effective in slowing down or stopping clots from forming in the first place. The way it works is to prevent the platelets from clumping together.

Be careful about taking a bromelaine supplement if you are on benzodiazepines, barbiturates, antibiotics or anti-depressants, as bromelaine will speed up the chemical processes in these drugs.

7 Cayenne pepper

Cooks often use cayenne pepper to add flavour to foods. This variety of pepper is extremely hot to the taste and is known as the 'King of Spices'. The main chemical in cayenne pepper is capsaicin, which gives the spice its fiery punch.

An online article from *Organic Lifestyle Magazine* says of this superb herb:

> While cayenne is amazing by itself, when it is combined with another herb, the results are worth more than the sum of its parts. Capsaicin helps every other herb function better because it stimulates the circulation of blood, which helps get the beneficial bio-chemicals and nutrition to the cells.
>
> Cayenne is an extremely effective treatment for heart and blood circulation problems, palpitations, and cardiac arrhythmia (irregular heart beat). It's a miracle for congestive heart failure and is beneficial for someone who has any type of circulatory problems, such as high or low blood pressure, elevated cholesterol, high triglycerides, and even varicose veins.

Among cayenne's wide range of health benefits is that the it contains is also an excellent clot buster, as it dissolves fibrin and prevents blood platelets from sticking together. A 2018 article in the *International Journal of Current Advanced Research*, 'A Scientific Review on Clot Dissolving Activity of Cayenne Pepper', says capsaicin causes the blood to flow properly through the blood vessels and helps to reduce the symptoms of poor blood flow, such as bodily pain, headaches, numbness in the hands, cold feet and leg tingling.

8 Cinnamon

The ancient Chinese and Indians used cinnamon for both culinary and medicinal purposes. And the fifth- and fourth-century Greek Hippocrates, known as the 'Father of Medicine', promoted the use of cinnamon in his medical treatments. The ancient Egyptians used cinnamon as part of their embalming process when mummifying their dead. The Romans also used it for medicinal purposes.

Cinnamon, a popular spice, comes from the inner bark of the *Cinnamomum* tree. There are two main types of this spice, Ceylon cinnamon and the far more widely used cassia cinnamon – the Ceylon variety costs more than cassia cinnamon. Both types contain the anti-clotting agent coumarin, the major constituent of warfarin, which can cause kidney, liver and lung damage when taken in large doses. However, Ceylon cinnamon contains 250 times less coumarin than the cassia variety, so is much safer to consume.

Coumarin inhibits the function of vitamin K, which, as we have seen, is an important vitamin involved in causing blood to clot. As cassia cinnamon is high in coumarin, it is used as an effective anti-blood-clotting agent. However, as with long-term warfarin use, cassia should be used with caution – you don't want to damage your kidneys, liver and lungs . . .

Norwegian researchers looking at how safe it is to take cinnamon – eaten widely in Norway – on a regular basis found that a safe tolerable daily intake (TDI), which means no adverse effects on health, of this spice is 0.07 milligrams per kilogram of body weight per day. So, a person weighing 145 pounds (66 kilograms) should consume no more than 4.62 milligrams of cassia cinnamon powder per day. This equates to less than a *sixteenth of a teaspoonful*, which shows how potent cassia cinnamon is as a blood thinner. To find out the exact amount of cassia cinnamon safe for you – with your body weight – to take daily, it is best to use a measuring scale rather than a teaspoon. Note: the Norwegian study just tested 'cinnamon', but we can safely assume this was *cassia* cinnamon, rather than the more expensive Ceylon cinnamon rarely found in products.

But be careful about drinking cassia cinnamon tea on a daily basis, as you could exceed the safe TDI.

9 Green tea

Black tea, commonly drunk in the UK, and green tea come from the same plant, *Camellia sinensis*. With black tea, the leaves are cut from the plant, rolled and then left to ferment, so they can be fully oxidized. When fully fermented, they are oven fired or dried.

With green tea the leaves are oven fired or steamed, to stop oxidation from taking place, and then rolled or shaped and left to dry. The process is shorter than that for black tea. So prized is green tea that it is the beverage of choice in Asia.

A 1999 study reported in the journal *Thrombosis Research* found that drinking green tea can prevent blood platelets from sticking together. A further study, in 2016, confirmed this, reporting in the *International Journal of Prevention and Treatment* that green tea can be used as 'a preventative strategy to lower the risk of thrombotic complications'.

So, how many cups a day of green tea should you drink? Research reported in the 1 January 2016 edition of the journal *Cardiology* looked at the effects of green tea on the cardiovascular (heart and blood vessels system) of subjects, as well as the issue of low blood flow through the vessels. The researchers investigated the results of nine studies on 259,267 people. They found the following:

• Those who drank 1–3 cups of green tea a day had a reduced risk of heart attack and stroke compared to those who drank less than a cup a day.
• Those who drank 4 or more cups a day had a reduced risk of heart attack compared to those who drank less than 1 cup a day.

Those who drank 10 or more cups a day had lower LDL

(bad) cholesterol than those who drank fewer than 3 cups a day.

The study concluded that consuming green tea benefits the heart and circulatory system.

Side note: while it's safe to drink 10 or more cups a day of brewed green tea, research has found that green tea *extract* (concentrated green tea made from the dry leaves) can cause liver damage.

Resveratrol

Resveratrol is a powerful anti-aging antioxidant found mainly in Japanese knotweed. It also exists in the skins of red grapes and in red wine. Other sources of resveratrol are dark chocolate, blueberries, cranberries and pistachios.

A 1995 study published in the *International Journal of Tissue Reactions* found that the resveratrol in red wine hindered blood platelets from sticking together and forming clots. The more resveratrol a subject took, the less the platelets clumped together.

To get more concentrated amounts of resveratrol than are available in foods, and thus increase its beneficial effects, it's a good idea to take it as a supplement. Resveratrol supplements usually come in 250 to 500 milligram capsules, and can safely be taken at dosages up to 5 grams per day. (A milligram is a thousandth of a gram.)

In the next chapter we move on to investigate an anti-clotting medical device your doctor may not have heard of.

References

https://www.drdavidwilliams.com/nattokinase-the-japanese-clot-busting-miracle (accessed 29 May 2017)

https://www.drsinatra.com/lower-your-blood-pressure-naturally-with-nattokinase (accessed 29 May 2017)

http://www.cleanmarinekrill.co.uk/krill-oil-vs-fish-oil (accessed 12 June 2017)

http://articles.mercola.com/sites/articles/archive/2017/02/20/astaxanthin-whole-body-benefits.aspx (accessed 12 June 2017)

https://www.ncbi.nlm.nih.gov/pmc/articles/PMC3249897 (accessed 31 May 2017)

http://jn.nutrition.org/content/131/3/951S.full?maxto (accessed 22 June 2017)

http://www.academicjournals.org/journal/AJB/article-full-text-pdf/7FE5DDC7506 (accessed 31 May 2017) http://www.greenmedinfo.com/blog/clone-if-you-fly-plant-extract-could-save-your-life-1 (accessed 12 June 2017)

http://www.bmbreports.org/journal/download_pdf.php (accessed 10 December 2021)

https://onlinelibrary.wiley.com/doi/abs/10.1002/ptr.6477 (accessed 30 November 2021)

https://pubmed.ncbi.nlm.nih.gov/11577981 (accessed 1 December 2021)

https://www.herbalgram.org/resources/herbalegram/volumes/volume-18/issue-7-july-2021/news-and-features-1/food-as-medicine-pineapple (accessed 1 December 2021)

https://www.organiclifestylemagazine.com/cayenne-and-capsaicin-natures-miracle-medicine (accessed 2 December 2021)

https://www.researchgate.net/publication/325597241_A_Scientific_review_on_clot_dissolving_activity_of_cayenne_pepper (accessed 2 December 2021)

https://www.sciencedirect.com/science/article/abs/pii/S0278691511006703 (accessed 2 December 2021) https://www.healthline.com/health/high-blood-pressure/best-natural-blood-thinners (accessed 2 December 2021)

https://www.livestrong.com/article/524042-can-you-take-cinnamon-with-a-blood-thinner (accessed 2 December 2021)

https://www.ncbi.nlm.nih.gov/pmc/articles/PMC4466762 (accessed 2 December 2021)

https://draxe.com/health/natural-blood-thinners (accessed 2 December 2021)

https://www.healthline.com/nutrition/ceylon-vs-cassia-cinnamon (accessed 2 December 2021)

https://www.mccormickscienceinstitute.com/resources/history-of-spices (accessed 2 December 2021)

https://researchmgt.monash.edu/ws/portalfiles/portal/303427439/303427373_oa.pdf (accessed 3 December 2021)

https://www.youtube.com/watch?v=Caq0AMr3f_s (accessed 3 December 2021) https://www.healthline.com/nutrition/how-much-green-tea-per-day (accessed 4 December 2021)

https://www.sciencedirect.com/science/article/abs/pii/S016752731500025X (accessed 4 December 2021)

https://www.drugs.com/resveratrol.html (accessed 4 December 2021)

https://www.mayoclinic.org/diseases-conditions/heart-disease/in-depth/red-wine/art-20048281 (accessed 4 December 2021)

https://www.medicalnewstoday.com/articles/resveratrol-benefits (accessed 4 December 2021)

https://pubmed.ncbi.nlm.nih.gov/7554275 (accessed 4 December 2021)

https://lpi.oregonstate.edu/mic/dietary-factors/phytochemicals/resveratrol#reference53 (accessed 4 December 2021)

https://pubmed.ncbi.nlm.nih.gov/7499059 (accessed 4 December 2021)

https://draxe.com/nutrition/all-about-resveratrol/
(accessed 4 December 2021)

7

Does your doctor know about this anti-clotting medical device?

*Science is the effective
way of doing things.
(Elbert Hubbard)*

A revolutionary leg pump

The Venowave is a device you strap on to the calf of your leg. It mimics the way the veins pump blood and replaces the need for compression stockings or blood thinners. However, you can also use it together with compression stockings and blood thinners, depending on your health situation.

The device weighs 270 grams (around half a pound) and needs two AA batteries to power it.

What conditions does the Venowave treat?

The Venowave has been developed to treat

• deep vein thrombosis (DVT)
• post-thrombotic syndrome (PTS), which is the after effects of having had a DVT (more on this below)

- lymphedema, where excess lymph fluid collects in the tissues and causes swelling
- varicose veins, which are the swollen purple veins that show through the skin (caused by damaged valves within the veins)

It improves blood circulation and lessens pain and swelling after patients have had surgery.

Is there proof the Venowave gets results?

Dr Ethan Light, in an article in the April 2010 edition of the *Venous Times* magazine, reports on a clinical trial that tested the Venowave on 32 patients. Of these, 26 were also using compression stockings and 26 completed the clinical trial. All of the subjects were already suffering from severe PTS.

PTS is the result of a blood clot lodging in a deep vein, which damages the vein. In the UK PTS affects between 20 and 40 per cent of people who have had a DVT.

Symptoms in the affected leg include

- calf pain (cramping or aching)
- a feeling of heaviness
- swelling (oedema)
- skin turning brown or red
- skin bruising easily, becoming dry and may peel

• rash

• painful sores (ulcers) that take a long time to heal

• varicose veins

And these can last for years.

The Venowave machine greatly outperformed the control device also used in the study, and Dr Light, quoting from the published abstract of the clinical trial, concludes, 'Venowave appears to be a very promising new therapy for patients with severe PTS, which may be used alone or in combination with graduated compression stockings.' He says that whereas earlier compression devices to treat PTS existed, the advantage of the Venowave is that it is less bulky, so it doesn't interfere too much with a patient's day-to-day life.

Also, the venowave.com website mentions a clinical trial published in the *Journal of Thrombosis and Haemostasis* in February 2012. This trial studied the efficacy of the Venowave in preventing DVT in 75 patients undergoing neurosurgery. The control group, which did not have the Venowave applied, also consisted of 75 patients.

Of the 75 who had a Venowave fitted, only 3 developed a blood clot, but in the non-Venowave control group 14 got a clot. This means the Venowave was effective in preventing a blood clot in 96 per cent of the subjects who had it strapped on.

Approved by the US Federal Drug Administration (FDA), Health Canada and the Australian government, the Venowave has entered the mainstream of anticoagulation treatment.

However, the Venowave is quite pricey, at around £300 in the UK.

Fortunately, there is a far more cost effective (and even free) way to keep your blood thin, one of my favourite blood-thinning methods. To find out what this is, see the next chapter.

References

http://www.webmd.com/dvt/tc/post-thrombotic-syndrome-topic-overview (accessed 7 June 2017)

http://www.e-dendrite.com/files/13/file/7VenousTimes.pdf (accessed 1 June 2017)

http://onlinelibrary.wiley.com/doi/10.1111/j.1538-7836.2011.04598.x/full (accessed 7 June 2017)

http://www.saringer.com/content/moduleId/UjWGmmW/pageId/Ty15HFIR.html (accessed 7 June 2017)

http://www.venowave.com/dvt-prevention.php (accessed 7 June 2017)

8

A powerful (free) way to thin your blood naturally

In all things of Nature there is
something of the marvellous.
(Aristotle)

Why blood gets thick

Human blood contains red blood cells, which make up about 45 per cent of the blood's volume. These blood cells have an electrical charge on their surface. If this charge is negative, the red blood cells get pushed apart, but if there is little negative charge, they clump together. This clump-ing makes the blood thicker and can lead to blood clots.

So, to avoid unwanted blood clots, it's important for the negative charge on the surface of the red blood cells to be high. And tiny particles, known as electrons, from the nucleus of an atom supply this negative charge.

How then can you keep your red blood cells negatively charged to stop them from clumping together? So your blood doesn't become like curdled milk?

A fast, natural way to thin your blood – and it's free

Where would you say is the biggest source of electrical energy (electrons) on our planet? A power station feeding energy into the cables of a large city?

No. The answer lies beneath your feet. The earth itself, with its enormous magnetic field, is the largest energy source you can tap into. If you can somehow connect your body to the earth's energy supply, you can take advantage of the oceans of electrons flowing through that magnetic field.

But how do you do this? Is there some complicated system to follow? Not at all. Every time you walk *barefoot* on the grass or sand, or take a swim in a lake or the ocean you are 'plugged in' to the electricity that comes from the earth's core. A steady stream of electrons flows into your body and keeps the surface charge of your red blood cells negative, so your blood stays thin and able to carry oxygen faster to your various body areas. Now you know why you feel so refreshed after a lengthy swim in the ocean, or after hours of walking barefoot along a sandy beach.

When I used to live in another part of the UK, I was constantly astonished when I went down to our local beach, about 10 minutes' walk from where Yvonne and I lived, to earth myself in the sea. So many people walking along the sand, but keeping their shoes on! If they only knew how health-promoting it is to go barefoot instead . . .

Is there proof a swim in the sea can help to keep your blood thin?

When I first heard about 'earthing', I thought it might be some kind of quackery, something strange people in a New Age cult might do. But light bulbs flashed in my head as I read about this astonishingly simple way to keep our blood thin and avoid further life-threatening blood clots.

One of the proofs that earthing is scientific, and not just the latest in a long line of health fads is a study conducted in 2013, described in the *Journal of Complementary Medicine.* Dr Stephen Sinatra, along with three other scientists, studied the effects of earthing on ten volunteers. The subjects had conductive patches placed on the soles of their feet and palms of their hands. Wires ran from the patches to a metal rod stuck in the ground. After two hours of earthing, also known as 'grounding', a small blood sample was taken from each subject and looked at under a dark-field microscope.

The scientists found that the negative charge on the surface of each subject's red blood cells had increased by an average of 2.7 – a leap of nearly 280 per cent. The study concluded:

Grounding increases the surface charge on RBCs [red blood cells] and thereby reduces blood viscosity [thickness] and clumping.

Grounding appears to be one of the simplest and yet most profound interventions for helping reduce cardiovascular [to do with the heart and blood vessels] risk and cardiovascular events.

Dr Sinatra says our blood should have the consistency of wine, not tomato sauce (ketchup). By regularly grounding yourself you help your blood flow optimally through your veins and arteries.

Another way to thin your blood – while you sleep

But how do you earth yourself when you're not able to walk barefoot outside or go for a swim in the ocean? Is there a way to be grounded while you sleep?

Yes. A highly effective way to stay grounded, even when you're indoors, is by using an 'earthing mat'. These are made of rubber infused with conductive carbon, and the larger ones (recommended, because you can put them to more uses) are 60 centimetres (24 inches) by 25 centimetres (10 inches) in size. They come with a cable and a special plug for the electrical wall socket, but you don't have to turn the wall socket's switch on for the earthing mat to work.

When it's time to sleep, simply place the connected earthing mat on your sheet below any part of your body, and go to sleep with the mat resting below you. Or, if you prefer, you can get an earthing *sheet* for your bed. Made of cotton, with conductive silver fibres, it fits over your mattress and has a cable that connects the sheet to an electrical wall socket.

One of the reported results of sleeping on an earthing mat is that it gives you a better night's sleep. I've found this to be true in my own experience. I used to sleep on an earthing mat, most nights, for about three years, and on and off since then, and believe it's one of the reasons I have not developed another deep vein blood clot.

Helpful if you work at a computer

Sitting for hours at a stretch working at a computer can be hazardous for your health. Dr Magda Havas, a professor at Trent University, Canada, has a shocking video on YouTube about the effects on her own blood of the electro-magnetic field around a computer.

With all electric devices around her switched off, she pricked her finger to get a blood sample. She then placed the sample on a glass slide and looked at her blood under a microscope. Some red blood cells were clumped together, but overall the clumping was in the normal range.

She then used her computer for 70 minutes before taking another blood sample and looking at it under the microscope. This time her red blood cells were 'sticking together like stacked coins', a phenomenon known as Rouleaux formation. Later that day she repeated her experiment, but this time with a cordless phone, which she used for just 10 minutes. Under the microscope she saw even worse cell clumping than when she'd used her computer for 70 minutes.

By earthing yourself with an earthing mat while sitting at your computer or speaking on a mobile phone you'll prevent your red blood cells from clumping together. One of the reasons why I got a deep vein blood clot, I believe, was because of all the time I'd spent working at my computer without a break. I'd sit with my legs bent under the desk for hours at a stretch. It's very unhealthy to do this, and it nearly cost me my life.

If you work at a computer, I suggest you use two earthing mats – one to sleep on and the other when you do computer work.

Cautions for warfarin users

If you're on warfarin, or any other blood-thinning drug, make sure you consult your doctor before starting to use an earthing mat. Because earthing thins the blood, if you earth and use a blood-thinning drug at the same time your blood could become dangerously thin.

In an interview with Dr Mercola, Dr Sinatra warns:

> I don't like people to ground when they're taking
> Coumadin [warfarin] . . . because we have had
> people ground, taking Coumadin at the same
> time, and their blood became like water.
> It was like red wine and then it got really thin.
> That could be dangerous.
> If you have high blood pressure, [or] . . . if you had
> a stroke and you have thin blood, it's a disaster.
> We basically tell people that if you're on
> Coumadin, you must work with your doctor,
> because your doctor's going to have to reduce the
> Coumadin.

A helpful book on natural blood thinning

To find out more about earthing and how it can help you
keep your blood thin, I suggest you read *Earthing: The Most
Important Health Discovery Ever!*, by C. Ober, S.T. Sinatra
and M. Zucker. This is probably one of the most important
health books I've read. It tells how its main author, Clinton
Ober, discovered grounding and how it transformed his
life. The book also describes how earthing greatly speeded
up the healing of cyclists who got injured during the Tour
de France cycle race.

References

https://www.youtube.com/watch?v=L7E36zGHxRw (accessed 5 June 2017)

http://articles.mercola.com/sites/articles/archive/2013/08/04/barefoot-grounding-effect.aspx (accessed 5 June 2017)

9

What to do if you have factor V Leiden

Nothing diminishes anxiety
faster than action.
(Walter Anderson)

What is factor V Leiden?

A mutation in the F5 gene causes the blood to clot more than it should. This condition is known as 'factor V Leiden', named after the Dutch city Leiden, where it was discover-ed in 1994. The 'V' is the Roman numeral for '5'. Because the F5 gene doesn't work properly, it's unable to turn off the anti-clotting protein C – which results in the blood over-clotting.

The F5 gene mutation can be inherited from either a father or a mother, or from both parents. If inherited from one parent only, a person who has the faulty F5 gene is five times more likely to develop a deep vein blood clot than the general population. However, if the faulty F5 gene is inherited from both parents, a person is eighty times more at risk of developing a blood clot.

What are its symptoms?

People who have the mutated F5 gene do not know they have factor V Leiden until they develop a blood clot. And they may never get a blood clot, even though they are more at risk than other people of developing one.

How do doctors diagnose it?

If someone develops a blood clot at a young age, the doctor may suspect that person has factor V Leiden. Or if the blood clot develops in an unusual part of the body – such as the spleen, liver or kidneys – this may be another pointer.

Doctors can use two types of test to check whether or not a person has factor V Leiden. The first tests how well the blood responds to the anti-clotting protein C. An abnormality shows the likelihood of factor V Leiden being present. The second test is a DNA test of the F5 gene itself to see whether or not it's normal. Both these tests are nearly 100 per cent accurate.

How many people have it?

According to the US Genetic and Rare Diseases Information Center, the following populations carry the factor V Leiden gene mutation:

5% of whites

2% of Hispanic Americans

1% of Native Americans

1% of African Americans

0.5% of Asian Americans

Also, up to 14 per cent of the people in Greece, Sweden and Lebanon are estimated to carry the factor V Leiden gene. So, the majority of carriers fall into the white/Caucasian population group.

Risk factors

According to the Mayo Clinic, people with factor V Leiden should be vigilant in the following areas.

Two faulty genes. People who inherit the mutated F5 gene from both parents are far more at risk of developing a deep vein thrombosis and pulmonary embolism.

Immobility. Long periods of sitting, lying or standing greatly increase the risk of a blood clot. This can happen during a lengthy plane flight, lying in a hospital bed during an illness or standing behind a counter while doing shop work. Because the leg muscles aren't moving, the blood isn't pumping through the veins and arteries as much as it should be.

Oestrogens. These are steroid hormones that promote female characteristics in the body. They're also artificially manufactured and used in oral contraceptives, or to treat menopausal and menstrual problems. Use of these can increase the likelihood in women of developing a blood clot.

Surgery or injury. Surgery, such as for a broken arm, or various types of injuries – say in a car accident – greatly increases the risk of an abnormal blood clot.

Blood type. People with the O blood type are less likely to get blood clots. Blood clots are far more common in those who have blood types A, B or AB.

Also, eating certain types of food puts you at higher risk of getting a blood clot (see chapter 5). And foods high in vitamin K should be kept to a minimum, as vitamin K causes the blood to clot faster (see chapter 2).

Ten vegetables high in vitamin K

The myfooddata.com website has a very helpful list of foods that contain a high level of vitamin K. I reproduce much of this info below for your quick reference – the list starts with the food highest in vitamin K and goes on to the food lowest in vitamin K. The measurements are shown in micrograms (µg). (A microgram is a millionth of a gram.) So, be especially careful when eating the vegetables near the top of the list:

1 Parsely. Per cup chopped = 984µg vitamin K

2 Kale. Per cup cooked = 544µg vitamin K

3 Broccoli. Per cup cooked = 220µg vitamin K

4 Brussels sprouts. Per cup cooked = 219µg vitamin K

5 Cabbage. Per cup cooked = 163µg vitamin K

6 Pickled cucumber. Per cup of = 130µg vitamin K

7 Asparagus. Per cup cooked = 91µg vitamin K

8 Okra. Per cup cooked = 64µg vitamin K

9 Green (snap) beans. Per cup cooked = 60µg vitamin K

10 Lettuce. Per cup = 56µg vitamin K

Ten fruits high in vitamin K

Below is a list of high-vitamin-K fruits, which you should eat in moderation if you have factor V Leiden or general blood-clot issues:

1 Kiwifruit. Per cup, sliced = 73µg vitamin K

2 Avocado. Per avocado = 42.2µg vitamin K

3 Rhubarb. Per cup, diced = 35.7µg vitamin K

4 Blueberries. Per cup = 28.6 µg vitamin K

5 Blackberries. Per cup = 28.5 µg vitamin K

6 Pomegranates. Per cup = 28.5 µg vitamin K

7 Blueberries (dried, sweetened). Per cup = 23.8 µg vitamin K

8 Red or green grapes. Per cup = 22 µg vitamin K

9 Prunes. 3 prunes = 17.9 µg vitamin K

10 Dried mango (sweetened). In 100g = 13.2µg vitamin K

Follow these two healthy diets to avoid more clots

There is no cure for factor V Leiden, as it is a genetic abnormality. But you can help yourself stay healthy by eating in moderation the foods listed above and adding other healthy foods to your diet.

In the online livestrong.com article 'How to Build a Healthy Diet when You Have Factor V Leiden', the author says:

> The best diet to follow is one full of foods that support heart health, because these are also naturally good for your blood health.
>
> Why? Heart-healthy foods help reduce inflammation and may help you get to a healthy weight, both of which are necessary for healthy blood, per Johns Hopkins Medicine. What's more, they can help lower blood pressure. That's important because high blood pressure can damage blood vessels, increasing blood clot risk.

The article writer recommends both the Mediterranean and DASH diets.

As its name suggests, people living in countries such as Spain, Italy and Greece follow the Mediterranean diet. This diet consists of fresh vegetables, fruits, nuts, seeds and legumes, as well as fish, lean protein, extra-virgin olive oil and red wine in moderation. Researchers have found that this diet is good for heart and brain health, fights inflammation and promotes weight loss.

According to the article 'Our Guide to the Mediterranean Diet' on the medicalnewstoday.com website, people on this diet avoid the following:

- foods made of white flour, such as white bread, white pasta and pizza dough
- refined oils, which include canola oil and soybean oil (rapeseed oil, while similar to canola oil, is more toxic and should also be avoided; see chapter 5)
- foods with added sugar, such as pastries, sweet carbonated drinks (sodas) and sweets (candies)
- processed meats, such as bacon, ham, salami, hot dogs and canned meats
- processed foods in general

The Mayo Clinic also recommends the DASH diet. 'DASH' = Dietary Approaches to Stop Hypertension – a diet that helps to lower or prevent high blood pressure (hypertension). High in potassium, calcium and magnesium, it helps to keep blood pressure in check. Foods high in salt, saturated fat and added sugar are kept to a minimum.

The Mayo Clinic online article 'DASH Diet' says studies have found that just two weeks on the DASH diet can lower a person's blood pressure. It can also lower the amount of bad, LDL, cholesterol in the bloodstream. 'High blood pressure and high LDL cholesterol levels are two major risk factors for heart disease and stroke.'

For eight years – from 2009 to 2017 – *U.S. News & World Report* voted the DASH Diet to be the best overall diet. It helps to lower blood pressure, fight diabetes and lose weight. The EatingWell website says the aim of the DASH Diet is to eat healthy foods rather than cutting out foods, such as carbohydrates, completely:

> The basic idea is to load up on fruits and veggies, choose whole grains over refined, include calcium-rich dairy items, and eat modest amounts of lean meat and fish. By including plenty of healthy whole foods each day, you naturally eliminate some of the not-so-great foods (like added sugars and unhealthy fats).

The EatingWell website presents a seven-day meal plan that follows the DASH Diet guidelines. Foods this plan promotes are, for example:

• eggs
• salmon
• chicken
• turkey
• hummus
• walnuts

- white beans
- avocado
- cucumber
- carrot
- sweet potato
- cherry tomatoes
- mushrooms
- pears
- apples (make sure these are always organic)
- raspberries
- clementines
- dried figs
- honey
- Greek yogurt
- cheddar cheese

In the next chapter, we look at frequently asked questions warfarin users ask.

References

https://www.mayoclinic.org/diseases-conditions/factor-v-leiden/symptoms-causes/syc-20372423 (accessed 11 October 2021)

https://www.mkuh.nhs.uk/patient-information-leaflet/factor-v-leiden-information (accessed 12 October 2021) https://rarediseases.info.nih.gov/diseases/6403/factor-v-leiden-thrombophilia (accessed 12 October 2021)

https://www.livestrong.com/article/282459-diets-for-factor-five-blood (accessed 12 October 2021)

https://www.ihtc.org/factor-v-leiden (accessed 12 October 2021)

https://factorvleiden.tumblr.com/post/50596598857/nutrition-vitamin-k-is-essential-and-healthy-for (accessed 12 October 2021)

https://myfooddata.com/articles/food-sources-of-vitamin-k.php (accessed 26 November 2021)

10
Frequently asked questions

Ask the right questions if you're
to find the right answers.
(Vanessa Redgrave)

In this chapter we take a brief look at five questions warfarin users often ask.

Is it OK to stop taking warfarin suddenly?

As we saw at the end of chapter 4, Dr Sinatra recommends certain high-risk patients should stay on warfarin to avoid developing further blood clots. If such patients stop taking warfarin suddenly, they may die due to a blood clot reforming. But lower-risk patients, in consultation with their health specialist, may decide to take the leap and replace warfarin completely with one or more of the safe natural alternatives listed in chapter 6. Plus, they may want to get a Venowave machine or earthing mat as well (see chapters 7 and 8).

What are the side effects of coming off warfarin suddenly?

As for the side effects of coming off warfarin? According to the drugs.com website, there are no negative side effects.

Again, though, warfarin users should exercise caution in stopping warfarin suddenly, and do this only in consultation with a medical expert.

Saying this, when I had a DVT, the 'medical expert' initially diagnosed me as having had a heart attack, even though I had no pain in the heart region and my right leg was red and swollen like a balloon. You might also want to be aware that, according to the 3 May 2016 issue of the *British Medical Journal*, the third leading cause of death in the USA is *medical error*! How wise is it to put your life in the hands of someone in a white coat, who claims to be a medical expert?!

How long does warfarin take to leave your body?

The website of the Western Australian government says it takes 'a few days' for your blood to become normal after stopping warfarin. And a doctor replies to a question on the steadyhealth.com website, 'If therapy with COUMADIN [warfarin] is discontinued, patients should be cautioned that the anticoagulant effects of COUMADIN may persist for about 2 to 5 days.' The medicine.net website says:

> If blood Coumadin levels are in the therapeutic range, in most people the effects are gone within 3–4 days of stopping the medicine.

If the Coumadin levels are too high (a toxic level), or a person needs urgent reversal of the drug (due to bleeding or a need for surgery), the effects can be reversed with injection of certain medicines to reverse the effects.

It seems then that around 7 days after you stop taking warfarin, all the rat poison has vanished from your body.

Is aspirin a safe alternative to warfarin or other blood thinners?

In a December 2016 article on Dr Mercola's website titled 'Is Daily Aspirin Therapy a Wise Choice?' he says, 'aspirin *slightly* decreases your blood's ability to form dangerous clots' (my emphasis). Mercola also cites a Swedish study that found aspirin can cause serious bleeding in some people. In the article he goes into great detail about the pros and cons of taking aspirin every day.

Dr Sinatra has an article on his drsinatra.com website titled 'Is Taking a Daily Aspirin Right for You?' He too warns that aspirin can cause internal bleeding and says, 'we must think twice about our overzealous use of aspirin'. However, he recommends daily baby aspirin for patients who have had a heart attack or for those who have heart disease.

Health expert Sayer Ji, on his greenmedinfo.com web-site in a 2015 article titled 'The Aspirin Alternative Your

Doctor Never Told You About', says Pycnogenol®, made from pine bark (see chapter 6), is more effective and safer than aspirin. Ji cites a 1999 clinical study that divided its subjects into two groups. One group received aspirin and the other, Pycnogenol®. The aspirin group experi-enced bleeding, while the Pycnogenol® group had no bleeding.

Ji also cites a 2002 clinical study that looked at the results of aspirin versus Pycnogenol® in a group of patients who had blood clots in the retinal vein of the eye. The results were clear. Of the 26 subjects taking aspirin, 6 dropped out of the study, due to the bad effects of the aspirin on them, and 2 of the 26 had bleeds in the eye. The Pycnogenol® group, on the other hand, had no side effects.

There are cheaper versions of pine bark extract than Pycnogenol® on the market. A search on the Internet (I use the startpage.com search engine) with the key phrase 'pine bark extract' should lead you to these (I buy most of my health supplements on Ebay).

I suggest you read what health experts Mercola, Sinatra and Ji say (see their articles listed in the 'References' section below) and then decide for yourself whether or not you should take aspirin on a daily basis, or instead perhaps use the safer pine bark extract or one of the other natural blood thinners.

I'm on warfarin for life – how do I cope?

This is a tricky question and there's no easy answer. As we

saw in chapter 4, long-term use of rat killer as a blood thinner can be deadly. Among its many side effects are that it causes hardening of the arteries, makes the bones brittle and can, in rare cases, severely damage the liver.

As I'm not a medical specialist, I point you again to the experts in this field.

Before listing some effective natural blood thinners, which low-risk patients can switch to, Dr Sinatra says patients in the high-risk category (see chapter 4) should stay on warfarin for life. He says this drug is 'the best preventative option for patients who are likely to experience blood clotting or stroke related to clot displacement'. As a stroke can lead to severe disability or even death, Sinatra's caution, based on over 35 years of clinical practice, is wise.

Side note: if you've found this book to be helpful so far, please *leave a review that says how the book has helped you.* I'd greatly appreciate it. Thanks!

References

https://www.drugs.com/answers/side-effects-coming-warfarin-after-warfarin-9-796733.html (accessed 5 June 2017)

https://www.bmj.com/content/353/bmj.i2139 (accessed 14 December 2021) http://healthywa.wa.gov.au/Articles/S_T/Stopping-warfarin (accessed 5 June 2017)

http://www.steadyhealth.com/topics/how-long-does-coumadin-stay-in-your-system (accessed 6 June 2017)

http://www.medicinenet.com/script/main/art.asp?article
ky =78970 (accessed 6 June 2017)

http://www.greenmedinfo.com/blog/aspirin-alternative-your-doctor-never-told-you-about#_ftn1 (accessed
6 June 2017)

http://articles.mercola.com/sites/articles/archive/2016/12/
12/aspirin-therapy.aspx (accessed 6 June 2017)

https://www.drsinatra.com/is-daily-aspirin-right-for-you
(accessed 6 June 2017)
https://heartmdinstitute.com/heart-health/coumadin-warfarin (accessed 6 June 2017)

http://www.wikihow.com/Live-with-Warfarin (accessed
6 June 2017)

http://www.ouh.nhs.uk/patient-guide/leaflets/files/
100429warfarinchildren.pdf (accessed 6 June 2017)

https://bloodclotrecovery.net/dealing-with-depression
(accessed 6 June 2017)

11

Side effects of five other blood-thinning drugs

Why are there never any good side effects? Just once
I'd like to see a drug commercial that says,
'May cause extreme awesomeness.'
(Unknown)

In this chapter I've used mainly the information found in the drugs.com website and have listed just fifteen possible serious side effects of each drug. To find out more about each of the five drugs mentioned below, go to drugs.com and search for answers to your queries.

Side note: drugs that deal with blood clots are either anti-platelet or anticoagulant in their action. The antiplatelet drugs stop the blood platelets from clumping together, while the anticoagulant drugs (also known as 'blood thinners') slow down the clotting process. Proteins in your liver known as 'cofactors' work together to make your blood clot. Vitamin K manages the creation of these proteins, and anticoagulant drugs stop the vitamin K from doing its work. Which is why, if you are on an anticoagulant such as warfarin, you have to be careful not to eat large helpings of foods rich in vitamin K, such as kale – too much vitamin-K-rich food hinders the effectiveness of an anticoagulant drug (see chapter 9).

Clopidogrel (Plavix)

Clopidogrel is an antiplatelet drug that cuts the risk of strokes, blood clots or serious heart issues. Fifteen possible side effects are as follows:

• blood pooling under the skin
• nose bleed
• bloody or black stools
• vomiting blood or small black bits that look like coffee grounds
• sudden severe headache that continues
• nausea and vomiting
• anxiety
• blistering and peeling skin
• pain or tightness in the chest
• joint inflammation
• seizures
• red itchy eyes
• swollen glands
• large swelling on the face or other body parts
• nightmares

Enoxaparin sodium (Lovenox)

Enoxaparin sodium is an anticoagulant and is a form of heparin (see chapter 3). It is used to treat or prevent blood clots and blood-flow problems as a result of angina and heart attacks. Fifteen possible side effects are as follows:

- bleeding gums
- coughing blood
- nose bleeds
- difficulty breathing or swallowing
- feeling dizzy
- headaches
- vaginal bleeding
- paralysis
- being short of breath
- blood pooling under the skin
- confusion
- convulsions
- fever
- extreme fatigue
- sudden fainting

Apixaban (Eliquis)

Apixaban is also an anticoagulant. It is used to prevent strokes and to thin the blood of patients with atrial fibrillation (a heart-rhythm disorder). It is also prescribed after hip- or knee-replacement surgery to prevent blood clots. Fifteen possible side effects are as follows:

- blood in the eyes
- blood in the urine
- bloody or black stools
- coughing blood
- nose bleeds
- confusion
- lack of mental alertness
- dizziness
- fainting
- constipation
- finding it hard to swallow
- joint pain
- nausea and vomiting
- sharp stomach pain
- tight chest

Dabigatran (Pradaxa)

Another anticoagulant, dabigatran, is prescribed to decrease the risk of a stroke that results from a blood clot due to atrial fibrillation. That is, atrial fibrillation which is not due to a heart-valve problem. It is also prescribed after hip-replacement surgery to prevent blood clots. Fifteen possible side effects are as follows:

- acid stomach
- black, tarry stools
- constipation
- diarrhoea
- nausea
- throat pain
- vomiting
- vomiting blood or small black bits that look like coffee grounds
- chest pain
- finding it hard to swallow
- losing consciousness
- unusual tiredness
- bleeding gums
- blood in the urine
- itching skin

Rivaroxaban (Xarelto)

Also an anticoagulant, rivaroxaban is prescribed to treat existing blood clots and pulmonary embolisms. In certain situations it may also be used to prevent blood clots. Fifteen possible side effects are as follows:

- bleeding gums
- bowel or bladder dysfunction
- numbness or 'pins and needles'
- coughing blood
- finding it hard to breathe
- dizziness
- vaginal bleeding
- nose bleeds
- vomiting blood or small black bits that look like coffee grounds
- arm or leg pain
- painful or burning sensation when urinating
- blistering skin
- irregular heartbeat
- vomiting
- severe headache

Conclusion

As with warfarin, the possible side effects I've listed for each of the above five drugs are serious. As soon as a person can safely stop taking any of those drugs, in my opinion, it is wise to switch to natural blood thinners that have no ill effects on the body or mind (see chapter 6).

Eight-and-a-half years (at the time of writing) after I had a life-threatening DVT and PE, I'm still alive and clot free – a living testimony to the effectiveness of natural blood thinners.

Along the riverbank . . . will grow all kinds
of trees . . . Their fruit will be for food,
and their leaves for medicine.
(Holy Bible, Ezekiel 47:12)

About the author

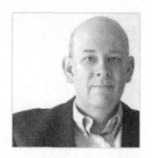

Former English schoolteacher Ed Barker is now a health researcher, writer and copy editor. He lives in North Wales, UK, with his wife, Yvonne. After his health scare and close shave with death in 2013, he started taking his health far more seriously – with special emphasis on exercise, an organic diet and weight loss.

In researching the deadly side effects of warfarin and heparin, he discovered safe natural alternatives. His research into other health areas also opened his eyes to the dangers of long-term use of pharmaceutical drugs, particularly to the liver. Since finding out how beneficial a gall bladder and liver flush can be, he has so far done six of these, with tremendous rejuvenating effects to his body. Try it!

Side note: if you like what you've read in this book and have found it to be helpful – please *leave a review that says how the book has helped you.*

Made in the USA
Middletown, DE
01 December 2023